Waltham Forest Public Libraries

This edition first published in Great Britain 2009 by
Crimson Publishing, a division of Crimson Business Ltd
Westminster House
Kew Road
Richmond
Surrey
TW9 2ND

A catalogue record for this book is available from the British Library.

ISBN 978 1 90541 052 1

Printed and bound by Legoprint SpA, Trento

Contents

Introduction

Of all the myriad childrearing issues that we parents face, getting the required quantities of good grub down the necks of our offspring can sometimes seem disproportionately challenging. Who hasn't, at some point, asked themselves concerned questions about the food their children eat? Questions such as: how many sweets are too many? Can they really survive on so little? And, just how long can it be now before scurvy sets in?

While feeding kids does come down to a fairly basic equation of good food + hungry child = healthy child, it's rarely that simple in reality. There are all sorts of reasons why children may not, cannot, or will not eat all the things we would like them to, and nourishing your offspring can be a fraught affair from the word go. Even when you've managed to establish what the good foods and the bad foods are, you must then strive to interest your little darlings in the former while encouraging moderation in the latter. And there's the rub: kids know how much it means to you that they eat the way you want them to. Which – often – is why they don't. It doesn't necessarily get easier with time, either. That unceremonious regurgitation of those early offerings of baby rice and pureed mango is just the start. Even when they're teenagers, and refusing to come to the table altogether because they'd rather just eat microwaved French fries from a box than move an inch away from MySpace, their eating habits are still cause for concern.

Truth is, there are some very sound anthropological and psychological reasons for the pressing need to feed we parents feel. Since the dawn of time, we've been programmed to ensure our children's survival and growth – and since those things cannot happen without nourishment, feeding them is automatically on the top of our to-do list. Right from the very start, moments after they're born and they nestle in for their very first glug of milk, the instinct to nurture and nourish our children is kickstarted. You could say it's basic human nature. The desire to get enough food down them – and good enough food – to ensure their survival is pretty much ingrained in us all.

All of which helps explain why there's something profoundly satisfying for a parent in presiding over a successful mealtime – whether a small baby hungrily sucking at boob or bottle, or a pre-teen devouring what's on their plate and then asking for more, it's always a huge relief to know your child is fuelled for at least the next couple of hours of their life – and why we worry so when our children's eating habits leave something to be desired, as they very frequently do. It can feel as though you're failing them on a fairly fundamental level.

Add in the fact that feeding kids has become a national obsession of late, what with the experts predicting a nutritional showdown ahead for the next generation of junk food addicts, and fears that the celebrity skin 'n' bone look provides an unhealthy influence the other way, it's hardly surprising that we fret so, while scraping the latest in a long line of rejected dinners into the bin. Food has never been more topical than it is right now. The nation's dietary habits and body issues are invariably headline fodder, with subjects such as childhood obesity, eating disorders, school dinners and our 'couch potato culture' always climbing the social and political agenda. It's no bad thing that these issues are everywhere – they are entirely in the public interest, after all. But it does add to the pressure and, at times, to the confusion, for parents who are already concerned about what and how to feed their children. (The answer is probably to take each news report or reality show with a pinch of salt – although, not more than your RDA of the stuff, naturally – and simply bear in mind whatever's relevant for your own family.)

We need to point out that this is not a book about eating disorders, although it does address the important question of when a child with food issues may be a cause for serious concern and/or need professional help. The vast majority of children who can't eat, won't eat, or don't eat the right things, can be helped with nothing more than the right support and attitude at home.

Experts usually advise panicking parents not to worry – reminding them that children will almost always eventually eat when they're hungry and even the worst of eating habits are pretty unlikely to kill them. This may be true, but it's hard not to worry when daily faced with an uphill struggle to get them to eat anything, compounded by the fearful knowledge that eating disorders, food allergies, and cases of obesity are on the rise among the nation's youngsters. Nowadays, it's hard not to be worried about what they put in their mouths, and how often.

Food issues of one sort or another are a perfectly normal part of family life, yet they can cause disproportionate levels of stress. This book aims to take that worry away by looking at the many and varied reasons for them, and outlining ways of tackling them. It also aims to take a broader look at how we can set up healthy eating patterns and – perhaps even more importantly – healthy attitudes towards food that will stand them in good stead for the rest of their lives.

This book has been written with the benefit of both experience and expertise. Consultant author Dr Sandi Mann is a mum-of-three as well a psychologist specialising in stress issues and author of several self-help psychology books, while Sally Child, a nutritional therapist with a background as a nurse and health visitor, has three grown-up daughters and a grandson. She lectures on children's nutrition and has written other books on the subject. Author Hollie Smith points out that she has no formal qualification in either psychology or nutrition, but she does have two young children whose difficult eating frequently drives her up the dining room wall.

It's true that you shouldn't worry too much about the way your kids eat. It's also true that you almost certainly will. The aim here is to help you find a happy balance between the two.

Nutritional information: What are healthy eating habits for children?

Why do we need to eat, anyway?

Just in case this isn't completely obvious: food is vital stuff. Its main role is the provision of energy, of which we all need a constant supply – not merely to fuel us in all our actions, but to drive the very basics of bodily functions, such as breathing, blinking, brain function, and blood circulation. Food also supplies all the essential nutrients we need to ensure our bodies are working, boost our immune systems, and to keep us in good general health. And it's crucial for development and growth – even as adults we still do a certain amount of this, because our tissues are constantly being replaced, but of course, it's children for whom the growth and development function of food is most relevant. Without food, they ain't gonna get any bigger.

🍅 Sally says: 'Children need lots of varied nutrients to help them develop. During normal childhood, especially early childhood, the body is in a state of constant growth, requiring more of the macro-nutrient building blocks offered by the major food groups, including protein and carbohydrates, as well more of the micro-nutrients we need that are found in vitamins and minerals. As a child grows, their requirements also change, purely as a function of increased size and therefore energy output. The main periods of growth and physical development are during

the first year of life and in the teenage years,
particularly around puberty, although growth spurts can
also occur at around five years.'

The basics of nutritional information

There's a huge amount of advice and guidance available these days on the subject of what constitutes healthy eating habits for children. Too much, sometimes, for those among us who aren't actually qualified nutritionists. But you don't need a degree of any sort to understand the basics of healthy eating, and how best to fit them into real life. Just a spoonful of basic research, and a pinch of understanding. That's why this chapter includes lots of practical information about the nutritional needs of children, as well as some sensible guidelines and tables, to help you along. We've also put sources of further information on the subject in the back of the book.

One of the keys to healthy eating is balance: getting a bit of everything from all the various food groups, in the right sort of proportions. Of course, this can be a challenge to say the least if you have a child who steadfastly refuses to touch anything from one or more groups or has an insatiable predilection for stuff from one or more of the others. We'll talk a lot more about those sorts of children as we get further into the book – for now, we are simply outlining the ideal.

It's unlikely you'll ever be able to dish up the perfectly balanced diet for your kids, so there's little point in trying obsessively to do so. But it's good to have an idea of what to aim for, and to know a bit about the different food groups, their roles, and what they comprise. That way, if you're concerned your kids are getting too little or too much from a particular group, you'll know what to offer as an alternative. Remember too that while it may be ideal, it's by no means vital to ensure that every single meal your child eats is balanced – if their general intake over the course of several days or even weeks features a good mix of foods, then that's fine.

What follows is a whistlestop guide to your child's nutritional needs.

PROTEINS

- Essential for growth and repair, enzyme and hormone production.

- Sources of protein are meat, fish, soya and dairy products, eggs, beans and pulses, wholegrains, nuts and Quorn.

- Ideally, protein should make up around a quarter of every meal.

Roughly speaking, an appropriately sized portion is the amount that fits in the palm of whoever's eating it. Obviously you'll have to guesstimate this sort of quantity, as you can't very well measure out messy foods like baked beans in the palm of your hand...

CARBOHYDRATES

Vital for the provision of energy. There are two types:

- Simple carbohydrates are found in foods such as white bread and sugar.

- Complex carbohydrates are found in foods such as unrefined breakfast cereals, wholemeal bread, oats and brown rice.

Needless to say the complex variety, which tend to be high in fibre, are the healthier sort (although it's important not to give the under-fives too much – their little digestive systems cannot cope with too much fibre, which may fill them up and interfere with the absorption of vital nutrients).

Kids need loads of carbs to keep them going – around half their diet generally should be carb-based, with a portion, ideally, included at every meal.

FRUIT AND VEGETABLES

Healthy and highly beneficial in many ways, fruit and veg contain fibre, which regulates blood sugar and is good for the digestive system, and a wide variety of essential vitamins and minerals.

> Most kids don't get enough fruit and veg – the official rule of thumb is to aim for at least five portions a day. Don't forget fruit is still high in sugar, so ideally they should get a good balance of both.

Five-a-day: What exactly is a portion?

If you're unsure about exactly what constitutes a child-size 'portion' of fruit or vegetables, the reassuring truth is that it may be a smaller quantity than you realise. Here's a rough guide to some of the most popular types – and how much, in an ideal world, they should be consuming...

(Children may need a little more or a little less than these amounts if they are a bigger or smaller than average height or size.)

FRUIT

Banana	Peach
1–4 years: small	1–4 years: $1/2$
5–7 years: small	5–7 years: 1
8–11 years: 1 small	8–11 years: 1

Dried apricots

1–4 years: 3

5–7 years: 4

8–11 years: 6

Plum

1–4 years: 1

5–7 years: 1

8–11 years: 2

Grapes

1–4 years: 8

5–7 years: 10

8–11 years: 12

Raspberries, blackberries and blackcurrants

1–4 years: 1–2 tbsp

5–7 years: 2 tbsp

8–11 years: 3 tbsp

Kiwi fruit

1–4 years: 1

5–7 years: 2

8–11 years: 2

Satsuma

1–4 years: 1

5–7 years: 1

8–11 years: 1–2

Orange, apple or pear

1–4 years: $1/2$

5–7 years: 1 medium

8–11 years: 1 medium to large

Strawberries

1–4 years: 3

5–7 years: 4

8–11 years: 6

Melon

1–4 years: 1 x 25g slice

5–7 years: 50g

8–11 years: 50g

VEGETABLES

Broccoli/cauliflower

1–4 year olds: 1 floret

5–7 years: 2 florets

8–11 years: 3 florets

Cucumber

1–4 years: 2–3 slices

5–7 years: 3–4 slices

8–11 years: 4–6 slices

Cherry tomatoes	**Peas**
1–4 years: 2	1–4 years: 1 tbsp
5–7 years: 3	5–7 years: 2 tbsp
8–11: 4	8–11 years: 2 tbsp
Cooked leafy greens (eg spinach, greens, cabbage, kale)	**Sweetcorn**
1–4 years: $^1/_2$–1 tbsp	1–4 years: 1 tbsp
5–7 years: 1 tbsp	5–7 years: 2 tbsp
8–11 years: 1–2 tbsp	8–11 years: 2 tbsp
Cooked pulses (eg chickpeas)	**Tinned or frozen fruit/veg, any sort**
1–4 years: $^1/_4$ small cup	1–4 years: $^1/_2$ tbsp
5–7 years: $^1/_4$ small cup	5–7 years: 1 tbsp
8–11 years: $^3/_4$ small cup	8–11 years: 2 tbsp
Cooked sliced carrots	
1–4 years: $^1/_2$ tbsp	
5–7 years: 1 tbsp	
8–11 years: 2 tbsp	

FATS

We all need some fats in our diet to be healthy, and children in particular need them to boost energy and growth – in fact, kids burn considerably more body fat than adults relative to the amount of energy they use, so they've got more scope than we grown-ups to eat and enjoy fats with impunity. There are also vital nutrients to be had in some high-fat foods such as dairy products (whole milk, yoghurt, cheese), and oily fish. However, some fats are better than others.

- 'Good' fats include the essential fatty acids, especially Omega 3 and Omega 6, which are important for heart health, skin, and brain function, and are found in nuts, seeds, leafy green veg and oily fish.

- 'Bad' fats are trans-fats (also known as hydrogenated fats and are often labelled as such – although there is no legal requirement for them to be), which are found in some commercial products, and can contribute towards blocked arteries, obesity, and may be linked to diabetes and so are best avoided. Saturated fats, which are found in fatty meats and animal products, pastry and many commercial products, are also 'bad' fats and should be eaten in moderation.

SUGAR AND SALT

Salt: How much is too much?

The RDA for salt, according to the Food Standards Agency, is a maximum of:

- 1–3 years: 2g a day

- 4–6 years: 3g a day

- 7–10 years: 5g a day

- 11+ years: 6g a day

Our bodies require a certain amount of salt in order to perform certain essential functions. But many of us eat more than is healthy – one recent survey found that most children eat twice the recommended maximum intake, probably because there's so much extra salt hidden in processed and pre-packed foods. The chart below illustrates how easily a child eating a modern diet could consume more than the recommended amount.

Salt content of some popular brands of typical foods:

Food	Salt per 100g	Salt per serving suggestion
Cornflakes	1.8g	0.5g per 30g bowlful
Sliced bread	1.1g	0.5g per slice
Cheddar cheese	1.9g	0.5g per 30g chunk
Mayonnaise	2.3g	0.3g per 15g dollop
Ready salted crisps	1.5g	0.4g per 25g bag
Breaded turkey shapes	1g	1g per serving of two shapes
Tomato ketchup	3.1g	0.5g per 15ml spoonful
Potato waffles	0.9g	1g per serving of two waffles

So, a daily diet consisting of a bowl of cornflakes for breakfast, a cheese and mayo sandwich with a packet of crisps for lunch, and breaded turkey shapes with potato waffles and a splodge of tomato ketchup could potentially add up to 5.2g of salt – well over the recommended maximum of 3g for four to six year olds, and just nudging past the 5g recommended for seven to 10 years olds. (And don't forget, the Food Standards Agency points out that these guidelines are recommended *maximums* – and that we should all in fact be striving to consume less!)

🍅 Sally says: 'Too much salt is dangerous for anyone, but especially children, as it stresses the kidneys and affects blood pressure. It can dehydrate a child quickly, especially as most don't drink enough. It also increases calcium excretion leading to weak bones and nervous system imbalances. And it's likely to lead to a lifelong preference for salty foods, which could mean an increased risk of heart disease, stroke and stomach cancer in adulthood.'

As a general guide, the Food Standards Agency advises that foods that contain more than 1.5g of salt per 100g, are considered high in salt, those containing 0.3g of salt or less per 100g is low, and anything in between is considered medium.

Tips for cutting back on salt levels

- Cook meals from scratch where possible, and leave out or reduce the salt you add, despite what the recipe may say. (Adults can add it later if necessary – but as we ALL ought to cut down on salt for the sake of our health, and should be setting a good example to our children, it would be far better if you didn't!)

- Instead of salt, add flavour with onions, garlic, herbs, spices, black pepper, or lemon juice.

- Don't add salt to the water when you cook vegetables, rice or pasta.

- Put limits on obviously salty snacks like crisps – keep these as treats to be enjoyed just once or twice a week rather than daily.

- Keep an eye on labels. Be conscious of foods that contain high levels of salt: ham, sausages, stock cubes, and certain breakfast cereals, for example. You don't have to avoid these altogether, especially if they also contain other useful nutrients, but it's a good idea to limit them to once a day. Bear in mind that some brands of packaged foods have higher levels of salt than others – so it's worth spending a few minutes comparing each. You'll soon know which ones to avoid and which ones to put in your trolley.

On food labels, salt content is often shown as sodium, but they are not quite the same thing as salt is actually a compound of sodium and chloride. To convert levels of sodium to those of salt, you need to multiply by 2.5g.

Sugar: How much is too much?

Sugar is also something we tend to consume too much of. Excessive sugar consumption can cause tooth decay, and is linked to obesity, early diabetes, and hyperactivity, so it's a sensible parent that keep tabs on how much of it their child is eating. As well as occuring naturally in many healthy fresh foods like fruit and milk, it's often to be found added in large quantities to commercially produced food and drinks (including a surprising number of savoury products), as the chart below reveals.

As a general guide, the Food Standards Agency advises that anything with more than 15g of sugar per 100g is high in sugar, that anything with less that 5g of sugar per 100g is low in sugar, and that anything in between is a medium amount.

More specifically, you might find the daily maximum amounts suggested here give you a good idea of what to aim for:

> **Recommended maximum amounts for a child's daily sugar intake (NB, these figures are averages: boys will need slightly more and girls slightly less.)**
>
> **1–3 years: 30g**
>
> **4–6 years: 41g**
>
> **7–10 years: 51g**

Do bear in mind that you don't have to banish something just because it has a high level of sugar – particularly if it is also a useful source of other nutrients, like yoghurt or baked beans, for example. Just keep an eye on the quantity they eat, and how often.

Sugar content of some typical foods:

	Sugar content in grams
Chocolate digestive biscuit	5.1g
Pasta bake sauce	⅕ of a jar, 5.8g
Cream of tomato soup	½ can, 9.8g
Baked beans	½ can, 10.4g
Mini chocolate swiss roll	12.4g
Slice of sponge and ice cream dessert	13g
Pot of white chocolate dairy dessert	14.7g

Fondant filled chocolate egg	25.4g
Blackcurrant drink	288ml carton, 28g
Cola	330ml can, 35g
Fast food chain cheeseburger and milkshake	41g

Sugar content of some popular breakfast cereals:

Cereal	Per 100g	Per 30g bowl
Frosties	37g	11.1g
Crunchy Nut Cornflakes	35g	10.5g
Coco Pops	34g	10.2g
Weetos	23.5g	7.05g
Bran Flakes	22g	6.6g
Cheerios	21.6g	6.5g
Shreddies	15.5g	4.65g
Rice Krispies	10g	3g
Corn Flakes	8g	2.4g
Weetabix	4.4g	1.32g
Ready Brek original	1g	0.3g
Shredded Wheat	0.9g	0.27g

Anything with 15g or more per 100g is a high-sugar food, so it's sensible to give these in small amounts, to keep them limited to no more than a couple of times a day, and where possible to give them as a part of a meal rather than in between, as snacks, as it's better for their teeth.

Tips for cutting back on sugar levels:

Be label-aware. There's no point in being obsessive about label-checking, or trying to calculate exactly how much sugar your child is eating – it would drive you mad and take up far too much time. But it's sensible, nevertheless, to have a broad idea of the sort of levels to aim for – and roughly how much they're consuming over the course of the average day. As the chart above shows, products like cereals can vary a great deal in the amount of sugar they contain – it's worth browsing a bit, and getting to know which are the baddies.

- When you're checking labels for sugar content, you'll find the figure you're looking for where it says: *Carbohydrates (of which sugars)*. It may display the amount of sugar per 100g, or the amount in one portion of the product, or both.

- Make cakes and other sweet treats from scratch where possible. That way you can cut back on the amount of sugar by halving what the recipe says (you'll usually find it barely affects the taste). And remember that pre-packaged savoury foods, such as pasta sauce from a jar, can also have a lot of sugar in them, so if you make this sort of thing yourself as much as possible you'll automatically be reducing their levels.

- Try to swap snacks containing high levels of sugar with nutritious alternatives. For instance, a chunk of cheese, a buttered wholemeal roll, fresh or dried fruit, or a handful of nuts or seeds are all better bets than cake, biscuits, or sweets.

⏱ Sally says: 'Too much sugar disturbs blood sugar levels, leading to cravings for sweet and refined foods, and ultimately causes diabetes. Symptoms could include irritability, bad behaviour, hyperactivity, poor sleep and an erratic appetite, not to mention tooth decay. Artificial sweeteners are even worse and some have been linked to cancer. There are a couple of healthier alternatives to sugar – one is Xylitol, a granular product extracted from tree bark which is just like sugar but with half the calories and a low glycaemic index (GI). You can just put it on cereals or fruit if needed, and replace sugar in recipes with it. The other is Agave Nectar – also a plant extract, it looks just like maple syrup or honey and like Xylitol it has lower calories and GI than sugar. It can be used on pancakes, porridge or with plain yoghurt. Both these products are available from health food shops and Agave Nectar from most supermarkets.'

Treats are fine... in moderation!

It's great to have a mental checklist of things that you know aren't good for them, and important to keep an eye on their consumption of these: the 'bad' fats, sugars and salt. But having said that, we are now duty bound to report that sweets and treats are an entirely acceptable element of a healthy diet, provided they are consumed in moderate quantities, and at appropriate times – that is, not before meals!

It's inevitable that children will enjoy stuff that's fatty, salty, or sugary. For one thing, it tastes great – how many adults out there can honestly say they don't harbour desires for one or more 'bad' foods? Also, these sort of desires go down deep: research shows that kids simply have an innate preference for sweet, starchy and high fat foods over fruit, veg, and protein[1], and with very good evolutionary reasons. Way back in time, babies who were crawling around in the wild, putting nuts and berries into their mouth as they explored, were at risk of being poisoned and so learned to associate bitter tastes with danger, while developing a preference for sweet (and therefore safe) tastes. And during periods of history where famine, disease and early death were ever-present threats, it clearly made sense to build up as many layers of fat as you could whenever possible. So it's hardly surprising that we have a lingering predilection for it.

Let's face it, you'd have a miserable childhood if you went without these things altogether – you might even end up being an adult with a serious addiction to them, desperate to make up for your years of deprivation.

However, the fact is, we owe it to our children to impose some kind of limits on foods of the 'naughty but nice' variety.

Aim to have sensible boundaries in mind when it comes to very high-sugar or salty foods like crisps, rich cakes, ice cream or sweets, especially if they have little else going for them nutritionally.

A good guideline might be to limit these sorts of things to just once or twice a week – in fact, some families find it makes sense to keep this kind of indulgence to weekends only. Try to give sweet things straight after, or as the dessert part of a meal, which is better for them from a dental point of view. And remember that plenty of foods are both nutritious and a treat: a homemade banana muffin; a bowl of plain popcorn; frozen yoghurt, or a few squares of good quality dark chocolate, for example, so aim to give these alternatives as much as you can when a treat is called for. As with so many things in parenting, it comes down to finding a sensible balance and then being reasonable, but firm, about it. There's more on this subject in chapter 5.

CALCIUM

Children need a good supply of calcium, to grow strong bones and teeth. It's recommended that:

Children aged 1–3 have 350mg of calcium per day, which amounts to:

- 100ml glass of whole or semi-skimmed milk +

- 80g of yoghurt +

- 15g of cheese

Children aged 4–6 have 450mg per day, which amounts to:

- 130ml semi-skimmed milk +

- 100g yoghurt +

- 20g of cheese

Children aged 7–10 have 55mg a day, which amounts to:

- 150ml of semi-skimmed milk +

- 125g of yoghurt +

- 25g cheese

Dairy products are certainly the most obvious sources of calcium, and just because your child doesn't like milk, cheese or yoghurt doesn't mean you can't get some other forms of these things in their diet.

For instance, try porridge for breakfast. It's a really healthy, often popular option, and sometimes kids don't even realise it's made with milk. There are loads of different commercial products, too, which might be worth trying, such as fromage frais and individual baby cheeses. (But do be cautious, as many of these products have a lot of sugar, salt or other additives in them, so you'll need to check the labels.)

Or how about trying to make some calcium-rich desserts at home, such as rice pudding, ice cream, chocolate *blancmange* or fruity cheesecake? These are also high in sugar, but the pay-off may be worth it if it's really their only reliable form of calcium.

Children under the age of two should always be given whole milk, as they need the full complement of calories. It's okay to give them semi-skimmed mild from the age of two, as long as the rest of their diet is balanced.

Also consider the less obvious alternative sources of calcium:

- Tofu (a 60g portion contains 306mg of calcium)

- Dried fruits such as figs (4 figs = 125mg of calcium)

- White bread (one slice has 64mg of calcium)

- Nuts and seeds (six almonds contain 31mg of calcium, while 2tbsp of sesame seeds has 130mg)

- Leafy green veg like broccoli (2 medium florets = 30mg)

- Oranges (75mg of calcium per medium orange)

- Pulses such as baked beans (100mg per 200g can)

- Canned sardines (about 250mg per serving)

Understanding nutritional information labels

There's a huge variation in nutritional value among what's available in the shops, and it makes sense to be 'label aware' so that you can tell at a glance what's in what, and make the healthiest choices – particularly as the information on labels can be highly confusing. These days, most of the big supermarkets have some kind of 'at-a-glance' system on their packaging to make understanding simpler and to avoid spending many hours of precious time flipping packets over and poring over the fine print during shopping trips. And when you've been doing it for a while, it starts to become more obvious which things can be bought freely, which are to be bought with circumspection, and which, on the whole, are to be avoided.

You can also buy calcium fortified versions of some products such as breakfast cereals and juices (check the labels though – the same warning about salt and sugar may apply).

If you're really struggling, you could consider an age appro-priate calcium supplement, available from health food shops and suppliers. Supplements aren't as good as the real thing, but for a short-term boost they're a lot better than nothing.

What, and how much, should children drink?

They're not strictly counted as a food group, but fluids are also a vital component of any diet as they aid the digestion of food and functioning of both brain and body. Not getting enough fluids can lead to dehydration, which can affect vital body functions such as digestion, energy and mood.

The amount children need to drink depends on their age and how active they are, but a good general guideline to follow is to offer six to eight drinks a day, in whatever quantity seems appropriate for their age group. For example, one drink probably amounts to:

- A small beakerful for pre-schoolers

- An average sized glass for a 6–9-year-olds

It may not be obvious if a child is dehydrated, but symptoms include irritability, tiredness, difficulty in concentrating and headaches.

Aim to give them a drink with each meal, and three to five others in between. In hot weather, or if they've been exercising, they'll need an extra cup or two on top.

> **Water is by far the best drink for children, with milk and diluted fruit juice fine in limited amounts (too much milk can spoil their appetite and fruit juice is high in natural sugar).**

Squash should be avoided or at least very carefully rationed as it's high in sugar and, unlike fruit juice, has nothing else in the way of nutrients going for it – if you do give squash, try and stick to one cup a day, make sure it's very well diluted (at least one part squash to nine parts water), and serve up only at mealtimes, when the affect of sugars on the teeth are reduced.

Drinks containing caffeine (tea, coffee, cola) should really be avoided altogether for children of all ages, because caffeine is a mildly addictive stimulant which can cause blood sugar levels to fluctuate, and the tannins contained in tea can reduce the absorption of important minerals like iron.

Consumption of other commercial drinks should also be carefully monitored. Many of these are marketed with the implication that they're a healthy choice because they're fruit-based, or because they boost energy, when in fact they may contain ingredients such as caffeine, large quantities of sugar, artificial sweeteners, e-numbers, and phosphoric acid, which erodes tooth enamel, reduces appetite, encourages obesity and decreases bone density. A quick check of the label should reveal exactly how 'healthy' these drinks actually are (for more on sugar and labelling, see below.)

> ✋ **Sally says:** 'My recommendation would be to avoid canned drinks and all other very sugary commercial drinks entirely, if possible, or at least to restrict them – for the over-fives only – to the odd special occasion. Even then, I'd sugest avoiding anything with sweeteners or caffeine in it. Fruit juice diluted with sparking mineral water makes a great alternative.'

How often should children eat?

Ideally, kids need three meals a day, served wherever possible at regular times: breakfast, lunch and tea (or dinner, supper, or whatever you call it in your house), with two or three snacks in between, in order to maintain their blood sugar levels – when these dip, the result can be a loss of energy, mood swings, headaches or poor concentration. A healthy but reasonably substantial snack is particularly important after school, when many children come in snarling like Mr Hyde, but fortunately can be swiftly transformed back to Dr Jekyll by the simple means of a fruit scone, a fruit smoothie or a flapjack.

It's also good to keep mealtimes and snacks regular and routine from a psychological point of view. If they know what to expect and when, they're more likely to be cooperative if you call them to the table, and less likely to demand extra snacks when they know it's too close to tea. And from a parental point of view, it just makes life a little easier and less stressful, too.

> **Breakfast is particularly essential for kids: it stokes up energy reserves for the day ahead and helps fuel their brains and boost concentration if they're at school. It also means they'll be less likely to crave an unhealthy snack later in the morning, and then spoil their lunch.**

It helps to be aware of healthy and unhealthy breakfast options, though – cereal and milk is a good choice, but of course, many are loaded with salt and sugar, so be selective (see the table on pages 16 and 20).

Include some protein in the form of milk, an egg, or yoghurt, and try and sling in a bit of fruit if possible so one of their five or more portions is ticked off early on (see the chart on page 12).

Home cooking is healthier

There's a good deal of pressure on parents these days to get into the kitchen and make meals from scratch. That's because fresh, home-cooked food is, generally speaking, bound to be healthier than anything that comes in a tin, packet, or plastic container with microwave instructions on the back – you know exactly what's in it without having to squint at the nutritional information panels. You also know what isn't in it, and that means artificial additives, colours, preservatives, hydrogenated fats, excessive quantities of sugar and salt, or any of those less desirable ingredients that lurk in many pre-packed and processed foods.

> If you like cooking and have the time and energy, our advice is to do as much of it as possible. And get the kids to join in too, if they will – naturally, it's a great way to involve and interest them in preparing good food and, in turn, encourage them to eat it, too.

If the thought of cooking from scratch makes you feel tired, it's worth remembering that it doesn't have to mean spending hours in a hot kitchen, shopping for hundreds of different ingredients, or trying to keep up with complicated recipes.

The culinary vogue these days is for simple food, fast, so there are plenty of inspiring cookery books around. And for the truly uninspired, many supermarkets now do a range of 'virtually' ready-made meals based around fresh ingredients that you can sling together at home.

However, it does have to be said that, often, the extra effort required to prepare something from fresh ingredients is very small:

> **A perfect example of an easily prepared fresh food is oven chips; real potatoes (scrubbed not peeled), tossed in a bit of olive oil on a baking tray, can be cooked in barely more time than it takes to slit open a freezer bag.**

Of course, many of us still need to, or choose to, use convenience foods on a regular basis. And that's absolutely fine – none of us needs any extra guilt and if the only thing you're fit for at the end of a long day is ripping the cellophane off a supermarket pizza, then you should be able to do so without feeling like a failure as a parent. When you do this, try and boost the meal's overall nutritional value by serving some raw veg appetisers beforehand, sticking a bit of salad on the side, or rounding it off with a piece of fruit.

"We run our own business and our working life, especially at the weekends, can be really crazy. We often used to dial out for an emergency takeaway, but we started to think twice about that when we realised that we can cook a fairly easy but nourishing meal in less than 20 minutes – which is the time it would take for the takeaway to arrive."

Farzana, mum to kids aged eight and six

Dr Sandi says: 'Convenience food, when you're stressed or in a hurry, is great and I don't think we should knock it. After all, we need to balance our kids' need for nutrition with our own need for sanity. It's only if you're giving it to them all the time that you need to stop and take a look at the way they're eating, because too much of it isn't good for their health.'

Sally says: 'I sometimes think mothers should have an extra pair of hands delivered with the placenta, rather than a lifetime of guilt. It's not easy, but the key to serving up home cooked meals is planning. Think about it the night before or in the morning and get ingredients out of the freezer if necessary to prevent the common scenario of getting to teatime and then not knowing or caring what you give them, as long as you give them something.'

An example daily diet for children

To help you put all the facts and figures into perspective, here's an example of the sort of healthy daily diet that's appropriate for a typical child aged 2–10 (portion sizes will vary according to their age, size, activity levels and gender). Stick to this sort of menu plan every day (allowing for the odd extra indulgence at the weekend, and a splurge here and there on holiday or for special occasions) and you can't go far wrong.

Breakfast

- Bowl of porridge with whole or semi-skimmed milk, sweetened with a spoonful of sugar or drinking chocolate; some stewed fruit, or a handful of raisins
- A glass of fresh orange juice, diluted with water

Mid-morning

- Piece of fruit +
- Glass of water

Lunch

- Jacket potato or wholemeal bread sandwich, pitta or tortilla wrap with tuna (mixed with a little mayo and yoghurt) or slices of cold, roasted chicken breast, or houmous, served

with a small bowl of baked beans, a side order of
homemade coleslaw, or a handful of raw veg crudités +
- Yoghurt or fromage frais +
- Glass of water

After school snack

- Glass of milk +
- Slice of malt loaf or plain sponge cake +
- Piece of fruit and a handful of almonds or pine nuts

Dinner

- Homemade spaghetti bolognese made with lean mince and
  lots of finely diced onions, celery and carrots, or for a
  vegetarian child, spaghetti with a plain tomato sauce made
  from finely chopped onion, garlic, celery, pepper, and
  carrots, cooked with a jar of passata or tin of tomatoes, and
  finely blended, with a handful of grated cheese on top +
- Stewed fruit, or small portion of fruit crumble with custard +
- Glass of water

Pre-bedtime snack

- Bowl of low-sugar oat or rice-based cereal and milk, or a
  slice of wholemeal bread with peanut butter +
- Glass of water or milk

In the end, providing a healthy diet for your children shouldn't be hard work, or a cause of much worry. Our advice is not to fret about every gram of sugar or salt, or to painstakingly take note of each biscuit or cake they consume, but to take a sensible overview of the whole family's lifestyle and try to make broadly healthy eating a normal part of your lives.

Summary

- Food is vital to our survival.

- We need a regular intake of something from each of the main food groups.

- Salt, fat and sugar are the three foods to be especially careful of.

- 'Treat' foods are fine – but best eaten in moderation.

- Homecooked meals are generally better for us than shop-bought ones.

- Regular meals and healthy snacks are important for happy, healthy children.

References
1 Wardle et al: Factor-analytic structure of food preferences in four year old children in the UK, Appetite (2001).

2

Starting early:
Why healthy eating begins
when they're babies

what this chapter covers:

- Try not to worry
- Set a good example from the start
- Weaning: why your baby's earliest experience of food matters so much
- Always aim to eat together
- Introduce different tastes and textures early on
- Offer plenty of fruit and vegetables
- Experiment with different flavours
- Is it okay to give my baby food from jars?
- Are distraction techniques a good idea?
- They won't miss what they haven't tried
- Why it's vital to remain relaxed
- What to do if you've started out badly

Parents can almost always save themselves grief, in many areas of family life, if they set up good habits and attitudes in the first place. And nowhere more so than in the dining room.

> **Research shows that how and what kids are fed in the early years of their lives can influence their eating habits and attitudes well into childhood, and beyond.**

You may well be reading this with your eyebrows raised if you are the parent of a small child to whom you dutifully fed a wide range of healthy foods from weaning onwards and who would eat everything you set in front of them until some point after their first birthday, when their interest in anything other than jam sandwiches and bananas went out the window.

This kind of behaviour is perfectly normal in toddlers, and there are very good reasons for it, as we reveal in chapter 4. For now, you will just have to take our word that it's usually a temporary phase and that establishing good, healthy eating habits when they're small will almost certainly make life round the dining room table a lot easier, later on.

⏰ **Sally says:** 'Broad tastes and good eating patterns are established very early on, and even if they're not obvious now, they will emerge later, when the terrible twos are past – or even later still, after the terrible teens!'

Try not to worry

It's not just the attitudes of our offspring that need some early attention – our own are all-important, too. Guilt and worry kick in from the start – let's face it, even in pregnancy we fret about what we're feeding them via the umbilical cord. Then once they've arrived, we become desperate to see that little arc on their growth centile charts go up and up. Heaven forbid it should go down!

It can leave a mum (or dad – but generally speaking, this is definitely mum territory) feeling that their child's failure to thrive is more about their failure to feed. It's one of the reasons the breast/bottle debate rages so heatedly – and why mums who struggle to breastfeed can feel quite traumatised by their difficulties. Perhaps if we could overcome the urge to obsess about these things when they're tiny, we might also be a bit more chilled about it all as they grow up.

Of course, it's easier said than done. But we're going to say it, anyway: stop worrying, right from the start. By all means seek advice from your GP if you are concerned. But in most cases, they'll be fine.

Set a good example from the start

The momentous period when you prepare your baby for a lifetime of solid food is also a good moment to assess your own eating habits and address any particularly undesirable dietary habits – if, indeed, you haven't already overhauled them while breastfeeding, during pregnancy or even while trying to conceive.

There's little point in spending hours slavishly creating healthy, varied meals for your children if, personally, you can't abide fruit, or you rarely sit down at the table for a decent dinner.

> **Your kids are watching your every mouthful as soon as they're old enough to sit upright in a highchair, and taking your lead. The business of setting a good example starts at the very beginning.**

Weaning: why your baby's earliest experience of eating matters

If eating habits are relevant from the start, then the introduction of solid foods is a highly significant affair for any parent. Unfortunately, it can cause a huge amount of confusion and concern as, somewhere between four and six months after they're born, our need to feed can go into overdrive, as suddenly it's about much more than just getting the required quantities of milk down them. Neither is it helped by the fact that – like so many milestones in a small child's life – parents often feel pressured by what everyone else around them thinks and does.

The matter of when and how to wean babies is subject to some debate.

Current advice from the Department of Health, based on guidance from the World Health Organisation, is that it's best to delay the introduction of solid food until a baby is six months old, because until then, their little guts are not entirely able to cope with it. However, both the Government and the British Dietetic Association acknowledge that some babies may need to be weaned sooner than this – although both emphasise that the absolute earliest you should consider starting is four months (17 weeks).

Because weaning is an important and potentially complicated issue, we've included some sources of further information in the back of the book.

Regardless of when you wean, the best thing you can do is to introduce plenty of different tastes and textures, gradually, but as soon as is viable. It stands to reason that if you give them healthy foods and a varied menu in the early years, they'll be more open-minded later on, when they've got a choice in the matter. But it's not just a matter of common sense – there's good medical evidence for it, too.

A 2005 study by Dr Gillian Harris, a clinical psychologist at the University of Birmingham, found that children's ideas about the foods they enjoy are formed early, and that babies exposed to a range of tastes, including fruit and vegetables, in their first year, went on to show a greater preference for them later on[1].

> Research carried out in 2002 by Skinner, Carruth, Bounds and Ziegler[2] suggests that by the age of two, children's food preferences tend to be relatively fixed for another six years or so – in other words, they know what they like, and they're going to stick with it for a while. So the more they're eating and enjoying before those preferences set in, the better.

Always aim to eat together

Research has shown (and it's pretty obvious, really) that if families eat together, around a table, it's a good way of encouraging healthy eating habits in children (and, for that matter, in grown-ups). Babies and toddlers are no exception.

> According to the National Literacy Trust, mealtimes offer a vital opportunity to boost little ones' communication and language skills.

It's a natural opportunity to model good social skills, too. Admittedly small children's hunger pangs may not always coincide with their parents'. But nevertheless, it's a good idea to pull their highchair up to the table and eat together whenever possible, even if it means you're eating earlier than you'd choose – or, if they really do need a much earlier tea than is practical for you, allow them to join you later, for finger foods or a snack supper.

> **Have fun, be relaxed, and talk – even if it's about nothing in particular. Show them from the start that eating is a sociable and enjoyable business. And this is advice that doesn't change, as they grow.**

Let them have a bash at feeding themselves as soon as they show an interest in doing so. But prepare yourself for lots of mess!

🍅 Dr Sandi says: 'Why do we have 'high' chairs that involve a baby being separated from the family at mealtimes? Babies should sit with the family. I love those chairs that allow them to sit at the table like everyone else – I think this sends a powerful message about the joys of food and eating, and helps them be part of the family.'

Introduce different tastes and textures early on

> **Aim to begin offering lumpy, thicker textures and appropriate finger foods one to two months into the weaning process – leave it too long, and they may balk when you do.**

This is a vital part of the process of weaning – as well as introducing them to new textures early on, they need food that's harder work to help their chewing and swallowing skills develop, and the development of speech. Be sure to supervise carefully, though, in case they choke, and offer new foods gradually, leaving three to four days in between to monitor for any allergic reactions. Once they've got to grips with textured solids, you can begin to feed them coarsely mashed versions of whatever the rest of the family's eating, assuming it's suitable* – as well as helping to broaden their taste and texture horizons, it's a lot less work for whoever's making tea.

---

*There are of course certain foods that must be avoided at certain stages in the first year for various reasons, and particular care must be taken if there's a history of allergies in your family. However, we don't have room to list them all here. This is by no means a comprehensive guide to weaning and you'll need lots more inform-ation at your fingertips if you're tackling it for the first time. Check out our recommendations for useful websites at the back of the book.

🍅 Sally says: 'Never add salt to cooking when your baby starts to eat family food. Use herbs to flavour and if 'die-hard' adult salt addicts still want it, they can add it to their own food separately.'

Offer plenty of fruit and vegetables

Include a wide variety of fruit and vegetables in their diet early on.

Puréed root veg – particularly sweet varieties like carrot or squash – or fruit such as pears, bananas and apricots are all ideal offerings at the start of weaning and after a couple of months they can eat most types of fruit and veg either cooked and mashed, or as finger foods.

🍅 Sally says: 'Berry fruits and tomatoes should be avoided before the age of one year, and citrus fruits until the age of one year, because they're not easily digestible and are more likely to trigger allergic reactions.

Experiment with different flavours

There's no evidence to show that babies prefer bland foods to highly flavoursome ones, and even if they seem disconcerted by a new taste, there's no reason why they can't develop a liking for it. Although it's true that babies have sensitive taste buds, their acceptance of different sorts of foods can be surprising (attitudes towards giving babies spicy food, for example, vary according to culture) and getting them used to unusual tastes means they're more likely to be receptive to them when they're older.

> **A few months into weaning, you can begin to experiment with different flavours using fresh green herbs such as parsley and coriander – as well as a good way to add interest, they're also rich in iron and calcium.**

Think broadly: consider sometimes offering them unusual foods even if you don't particularly like them yourself – for example, avocado, quinoa, or tropical fruits. And keep trying – even if they reject a food the first time, wheel it out again a bit later as there's every chance they'll change their mind.

Is it okay to give my baby food from jars?

Baby food in jars tends to be blander than fresh equivalents, and many of them contain undesirable extra ingredients such as sugar or starch, which is used to bulk out commercial foods and often contains wheat, which is best avoided before nine months, in case of allergies. Some are better than others so if you're swayed by the convenience of them, be careful about reading the label and look for those with the most natural ingredients. Aim to make jars occasional rather than the norm, though – homemade really is tons better for babies.

> **Making homemade baby food doesn't have to mean much extra work if you just portion off a bit of what the rest of the family's eating and serve appropriately.**

Once they're past their first birthday, you won't even need to mash it. You do of course have to pay careful regard to how much salt and/or sugar is in it as both these things should be avoided for babies under the age of one. Serving their food this way is less hassle for you, and a great way to introduce them to normal, healthy eating habits.

> **Fresh, high-quality shop-bought baby foods can of course be a great alternative when you just don't have the time, and in fact there are some very good ones available now in the chiller cabinets, such as Organix, Ella's Kitchen, or Little Dish, so if you're checking the labels and you're satisfied with what's in them, carry on.**

🍅 **Sally says:** 'Commercial baby foods often have added ingredients which means there's simply less space for the good stuff. Some companies use corn syrup, for example, which is just a form of sugar. When you make your own, you know it's pure and fresh. Recently, however, several companies have begun selling really natural, organic, fresh baby foods with no nasties inside them. Look in the chiller cabinets and check out the labels before you buy.'

Are distraction techniques a good idea?

Don't force or push them to eat anything they clearly don't want to. And don't go overboard on 'distraction techniques' such as pretending the spoon is a train and their mouth is a tunnel. That kind of thing's fine if it really helps get the grub in, but you don't want it to become so habitual that it's the only way they'll ever eat their dinner.

🍅 **Dr Sandi says:** 'I've sometimes resorted to using distraction when it comes to feeding my own children, but there are limits! I think once we start fighting them, or trying too hard, we get into power struggles and that's something you don't want to do with food, ever. So, if your baby refuses food, by all means try distraction techniques (getting daddy to make faces or a sibling to sing a song but if it's not helping much, forget it.'

They won't miss what they haven't tried

Babies who haven't hit their first (or even second) birthday really don't need anything in the way of edible treats – they won't miss what they don't know! Although there's a huge amount of joy to be gained from seeing the look on their face when their first ever chocolate button explodes on their tongue, aim to push this inevitable milestone back as long as you reasonably can. It's harder with siblings around, of course – wherever possible, distribute treat foods to older children when the little one's asleep, or elsewhere.

Once you've gone there (and let's face it, there's no turning back), keep chocolate, sweets, cake, and sugary biscuits for babes and toddlers carefully limited. Be prepared to ward off hunger pangs whenever they arise by keeping supplies of healthy alternative snacks like rice cakes, bread sticks and fruit on you at all times.

> Be careful not to fall into the trap early on of giving treats either as comfort, bribery or reward, because they will start to associate those foods with all those things and come to expect them every time.

It's never too early to start encouraging healthy eating habits in children. Naturally, it's so much easier to set up preferences for healthier foods from the start, rather than trying to overhaul unhealthy eating habits later, when they're thoroughly entrenched.

🍎 **Dr Sandi says:** 'Many parents are tempted to offer chocolate and other treat foods to babies because of their own agenda – they know how much pleasure there is to be had in them and they want to share that enjoyment with their little ones. But there's no real reason for introducing chocolate and other treat foods to a baby's diet – until they're old enough to know those things are out there, they won't know what they're missing. Babies and toddlers are generally thrilled to get rice cakes or fruit, so why give them rubbish instead? It's true that it's much easier to delay their introduction if there aren't older brothers and sisters around. My firstborn thought raisins were the bee's knees in terms of treats until she was about three; my second learned earlier about the joys of chocolate. Babies want what everyone else has and there's no point giving them the same meals but different snacks – they won't like that. The solution is to give the older ones their 'unhealthy' snacks when the baby's asleep, or better still, to cut down on their goodie intake, too. Make a big deal about siblings sitting down and sharing the baby's bananas or breadsticks sometimes.'

Why it's vital to remain relaxed

Aim to be relaxed and positive about food and mealtimes right from the start. It's a worry when babies and toddlers won't eat – not to mention annoying, especially if you've made a special effort to prepare what you've offered them. But it's really important not to show them you care. They'll be picking up on that kind of feedback before they've even picked up their own spoon.

> ☁ Dr Sandi says: 'Babies have little control over their lives – they're picked up, changed, plonked down, handed over. As they develop they start to exert their own sense of self and that means trying to exert their will. They do this by engaging in power struggles: screaming when they object to being put in the bath, arching their back if they don't want to be forced in their buggy, and clamping their mouths shut when you try to feed them. Don't get into mealtime battles. Stay calm, try again a little later, or hang back and allow them to feed themselves for a while.'

What to do if you've started out badly

If you're reading this and feel that you're probably broken every bit of advice we've given, don't panic. In the following chapters, we not only discuss how to instil healthy eating habits into your difficult eater, but also how you can undo some of the groundwork. Turn to chapter 5 for practical advice on how to start right now.

Summary

- How and what they eat from the start will influence their eating habits later.

- Offer babies a wide variety in tastes and textures early on in life.

- The importance of parental attitudes begins early on, too.

- It's never too early to encourage healthy eating.

- Give babies their meals with the whole family whenever possible – it passes on important messages about food and eating as a pleasurable, sociable thing.

References

1 Greville-Harris: Towards an understanding of how young children make and overcome neophobic food responses, (2004).

2 Skinner, Carruth, Bounds and Ziegler: Children's Food Preferences: A Longitudinal Analysis, (2002).

3

Your input:
The importance of setting a
good example

what this chapter covers:

- Attitudes to eating are laid down early in life
- Why you need to eat your greens too
- Why we should eat our meals at the table
- Enjoying the same meal, together
- How to make your children 'foodies'
- Get the balance right

Attitudes to eating are laid down early in life

If we want our kids to have good eating habits and a healthy attitude towards food, then of course, it's largely down to us to pass those things on. It's pretty obvious, really, but parental attitudes and examples are absolutely crucial when it comes to food and feeding – as indeed they are to every aspect of bringing up children.

Take a moment to think back to your own childhood. Chances are, you can pinpoint a great many ways that your existing food habits and attitudes were set up for life by your earliest influences – for better or worse. Maybe you were forced to eat something you didn't like, and now you hate it. Perhaps chocolate was hugely significant, so these days you struggle to get through an evening without some. Possibly you never sat down for a meal with your family, and you can't particularly see the point of doing so now.

> **The eating habits we lay down during our kids' childhoods – consciously or otherwise – are likely to affect their eating habits as an adult.**

A heavy responsibility, it's true. But the simplest, healthiest way to bear it is by setting the right example, practically and emotionally, as far as we possibly can. There's nothing to be lost by doing so: in fact, our own health stands to benefit, too.

Why you need to eat your greens, too

As we've mentioned, there are lots of reasons – some of them intrinsically tied up with our own childhoods and early relationships – why many adults have one or more food-related 'issues' of their own.

Plenty of grown-ups, for example, are fussy eaters, or simply cannot abide certain foods (and let's face it, it's a rare person who'll eat anything set in front of them). Not all of us are necessarily good at eating our greens. And who among us doesn't lean towards a craving for chocolate, crisps, or some other sort of 'unhealthy' food? These are all pretty normal tendencies (it is, after all, basic biology to crave fat and sugar in case we should ever get caught up in a famine) and, assuming they are not excessive or out-of-control habits that may be affecting your health, and that the rest of your diet is a reasonably 'balanced' one, nothing to beat yourself up about.

> If there's a rather extreme element of your diet that you know leaves a lot to be desired, you either need to work out ways of keeping it from your kids, or you need to work on ways of overcoming it.

Needless to say, it's better all round if you can aim for the second of those two. Shoving Mars Bars into your mouth to satisfy your desperate, daily need for chocolate when they're not looking isn't a very emotionally healthy way to behave.

And anyway, you're sure to be rumbled. Kids can smell the stuff on your breath at 20 paces.

"I adore chocolate, and I have to have some every day. I know it's probably not a great food habit for my kids to see, so I usually try and save my fix for after bedtime or when they're at school. It seems a bit deceitful, but I figure what they don't know won't affect them. And anyway, I'm a grown-up – I like to think I can keep my cravings under control! We also eat it together sometimes, on a more occasional basis. They love chocolate at least as much as I do, but they know it's a treat and not something, ideally, to be munched on every day of the week.**"**

Rachel, mum to kids aged nine, seven and three

🍅 **Dr Sandi says:** 'Always bear in mind the old maxim, "Do as I say not as I do". Often parents eat things that they won't allow their kids, with the excuse that "I'm an adult, I am allowed". This sends mixed messages and just makes kids long to be able to make their own unhealthy choices like you. So, unless you can be sure they won't find out, don't eat anything that you don't want them to know about.'

Eating out

Eating out once in a while can be a good chance to experiment, as well as a fun thing to do as a family. A change of scenery is a good way to relieve the pressure if things sometimes get a little heated in your own dining room, and children are often swayed into experimenting by the sheer novelty value of a restaurant meal, particularly if the various features of a completely different culture are involved: chopsticks, hot flannels, or sizzling fajitas brought to your table, for instance, may well tempt little appetites – as long as it's not an establishment that peddles nothing but junk food, of course.

> If you're not a great experimenter of different foods yourself, perhaps now's the time to start trying.

🍅 Sally says: 'Meals out are a good way to broaden their experiences. If the children's menu leaves something to be desired, ask for a small or half portion of what's on offer for the adults, instead.'

Why we should eat our meals at the table

Busy lives are par for the course these days, and families are commonly fragmented by different interests and schedules. But even so, it's a great shame that the habit of eating together at the table has lapsed to such an extent.

> **Some fairly shocking research suggested that as few as three in 10 families sit down together more than once a week.**
> **(Source: 2004 National Family Mealtimes Survey, by the Raisingkids website)**

A whole raft of research has found reasons why it's a good idea for families to eat together at the table whenever possible:

- It strengthens relationships and boosts communication.[1]

- It encourages conversation and increases linguistic abilities.[2]

- It helps teens cope with the stresses of adolescence.[3]

- It reduces the likelihood of adolescent girls adopting extreme dieting methods later on.[4]

- It helps to pass on good attitudes about food and good table manners.[5]

- It leads to better nutrition.[6]

But scientific findings aside, it stands to reason that sitting down and taking your time over meals so that they're regular, relaxed, and sociable events is likely to enhance the whole family's enjoyment and acceptance of good food. Even if you can't do it daily, perhaps because your working hours don't allow, or because it's rare for all adults and children in your home to be present and correct at the same time, aim to make it a habit at the weekends, at least.

Of course, some people quite rightly point out that family mealtimes are not always the idyll that's painted by the experts, or even a particularly practical option for many modern families. The aim is to make mealtimes enjoyable, so don't force it, especially if your dining room is commonly a scene of conflict, or the stress of trying to get everyone sitting down and eating the same things is becoming a pressure you could do without.

> **If your family isn't used to sitting down together much, introduce the habit, or increase the number of occasions you do so gradually.**

Try upping the interest stakes by serving up a universally popular meal or laying the table in a funky way – for special occasions you could get the kids to make placemats, napkin holders, place names, or menu cards.

Enjoying the same meal, together

Aim to eat the same meal, whenever possible. This helps to reinforce the message that they've got to keep on trying what's put in front of them, and is also, of course, an awful lot easier on whoever's in charge of catering. Of course, you have to be realistic and flexible about it, especially if you've got one or more fussy eaters on your hands, so aim to provide base meals which you can easily adapt to suit more than one preference. For example if if you're making a curry, save the spicy additions until later if they really can't do the hot stuff.

> **With most meals, there's almost always a kid-friendly version that can be rustled up with a little thought and effort.**

You're no one's slave – but a certain amount of indulgence may be required.

How to make your children 'foodies'

Food is a glorious thing! And not just because it keeps us alive – if it tastes good it can make us feel fabulous, and if we eat with other people it can be a wonderfully cohesive social experience. Foster your kids' interest in (good) food by encouraging them to help you plan, cook or prepare meals, and shop for it together.

> **Talk about food, whenever you get the chance – how good it tastes, where it comes from, and how it benefits us.**

Children of all ages usually love to don an apron and get cooking. There are loads of kids' cookery books on the market, but even if you can't quite find the time and energy to guide them through fairly complex recipes (or you don't think you can face the mess it will involve), they'll still love to be involved in the preparation of simple snacks (such as pizzas, muffins with toasted cheese and tomato, eggy bread, easy dips, and fruit salad) and, hopefully, in the eating of them, too.

> **Growing your own is a great way to boost their interest in, and liking for, fruit and vegetables.**

If you don't have green fingers, or much in the way of a garden, you can still cultivate herbs, tomatoes and salad vegetables in a pot or on a windowsill pretty easily. In the summer months, a trip to a pick-your-own farm is always good fun – even hardened fruit-avoiders may be tempted by juicy, sweet strawberries plucked direct from the plant, or peas popped straight from the pod. And even the humble supermarket is a good place to interest them in fresh fruit and veg (if you can bear to take them – and lots of parents can't). Let them select what they want to try – if they've got one of those machines that weighs produce and spits out a sticker, so much the better. They'll be more likely to be receptive if they've made their own choices.

Get the balance right

Of course, you can have too much of an interest in a healthy lifestyle. It's great for your children to see you dishing up and eating a balanced diet as a matter of course. And it's good if they have a basic understanding of which foods are healthy and why, and which things are to be enjoyed in a more moderate way. But pushing a healthy lifestyle down their throats is a sure way to make a child feel isolated and unusual.

> Let's face it, who'd want to be one of those poor little kids whose mother brings out a bag of carrots at parties and takes the plate of chocolate fingers out of their reach?

Children really don't need an influential adult hovering over them who constantly obsesses or frets about what they're eating. Banging on incessantly about 'good' and 'bad' foods could cause them to form associations with them in their minds and, more profoundly than that, may instill in them either an overwhelming desire for, or an extreme aversion to unhealthy foods, which in years to come may develop into a serious psychological issue for them, possibly even an eating disorder. In fact, there's growing concern among experts and commentators that the current healthy eating and anti-obesity drive may result in the unwanted backlash of increasing eating disorder statistics among youngsters. So clearly, a chilled-out approach is what's needed.

The key is taking a holistic approach to good health, and finding a happy balance – if they eat well the majority of the time and live an active life, there'll be plenty of scope for the 'naughty' stuff to be enjoyed in sensible quantities. (Be sure to avoid calling it 'naughty', though, or you may inadvertently boost its appeal.)

As for calorie-counting and weight-loss programmes, well, that really isn't a happy example for an adult to be setting a child – especially 'yo-yo' dieting, a constant striving and failure to lose weight. If you're dieting for the sake of your health, be really honest and explain why it is you are doing it. This will reinforce the importance of healthy eating to your child, and you will be a great example to them.

Diets don't often work in the long term, anyway: and the best approach to losing weight is to make small, achievable, and permanent changes to your lifestyle so that you eat well and keep active all the time. If you do it this way, your family probably won't even notice that you're on a 'diet'.

66 There's been a lot of emphasis on healthy eating at her school recently, and my little girl's started coming home and saying, 'we can't eat that Mummy – it's bad for you'. I think it's right that they learn this stuff, but it worries me a bit. I'd hate for her to start obsessing. So I tell her there's no such thing as bad food, everything's okay once in a while. 99

Theresa, mum to a daughter aged six

❝I lost almost three stone last year on a diet programme and I did seriously consider what the children were likely to think before I started. I didn't want them to think that 'skinny' was desirable and that 'fat' was wrong. I never called it a diet and I made sure that we sat together at mealtimes just as normal, so that they didn't think I was starving myself, and we'd talk about losing weight for me as being a healthy thing, and so that I could have more energy. During the programme, I learned a lot about healthy food, so I can honestly say that overall we as a family eat a lot more healthily now.**❞**

Farzana, mum to kids aged eight and six

Summary

- If we want our kids to be good eaters, we have to be good eaters too. But that's a good thing – it means we'll be healthy, as well.

- Make healthy eating part of the whole family's lifestyle.

- If you have any negative issues with food yourself, you should sort them out.

- Offer as much choice and variety as you can get away with.

- Eat together.

- Help them to appreciate eating as the positive experience it should be.

- Don't go overboard and don't obsess. Balance is everything.

- Watch your language. Be mindful of what you say about food in front of your children.

References

1 Focus Group Report by Nancy Lee, Nutrition Education Network of Washington, (July, 1996).

2 Using 'rare' words at mealtime can enlarge children's vocabulary by Carolyn Sanford.

3 Suppers on! Adolescent adjustment and frequency of family mealtimes by Bowden and Zeisz, (1997).

4 Project EAT, Dianne Neumark-Sztainer, University of Minnesota School of Public Health.

5 Is Family Mealtime Important? by Leah Davies.

6 Harvard Study pub. Archives of Family Medicine, (March, 2000).

Why are some children difficult eaters?

Fussy eating: a very normal childhood phase

There are all sorts of reasons why children of all ages decide they can't, or won't, eat what's put in front of them. Although sometimes complex, most of these reasons are normal and, in spite of what our instincts as nurturers and nourishers dictate, nothing to be seriously worried about.

If taken to its very extremes, or if it goes on for long enough, selective or fussy eating may require some professional help. But the truth is, things have to be pretty bad to get to that point.

> For the most part, selective or fussy eating is a normal but temporary developmental phase which rarely becomes dangerous to health. It's quite fair to say that the vast majority of children will go through it at some level, and at some point in their lives.

Why are some children fussy eaters?

Some children are selective eaters from the start, as a result of difficulties during weaning – often caused by medical problems such as food intolerance or allergies. But most parents find it kicks in later. Very often, a child eats enthusiastically after weaning, then ceases to do so some time between their first and second birthdays. This tendency is extremely common, and there are a number of likely reasons for it.

Primary among them is what the experts call neophobia, literally meaning 'fear of new foods'. It's believed there may be very good evolutionary reasons for neophobia, namely that babies have developed a suspicion of strange foods because it was necessary for their ancestors to steer clear of anything poisonous. Hence they can reject or appear to be disgusted by something before they've even put it in their mouths. Fortunately, neophobic tendencies tend to phase out over time, as it begins to dawn on them that people around them are eating different foods without keeling over.

Some children are simply more neophobic than others. Research suggests that while environmental factors may also be significant, it's probably genetic – in other words, inherited from their folks[1].

Another theory is that kids may become more selective as toddlers because they're starting to develop memories and they begin to realise that each meal is not their last – they know full well that they'll be getting fed again later. Not only that, they quickly learn that better things might be around the corner – even if not at home with you, then round at a friend's house or during snack time at toddler group. They also know that if they complain they are hungry later, they may well be offered something that's nicer than what's on their plate right now.

Psychology undoubtedly plays its part, too. Once they're old enough to know how, toddlers are constantly looking for ways to exercise what little power they have over the adults around them and, as they learn all about the joys of independence, are keen to put it into practice.

> **Toddlers like to push boundaries and to gently poke at adult patience levels, just to see how much scope they've got before they finally provoke a blown gasket.**

And of course, kids of all ages can be gold medal attention-seekers. Where better to indulge in all these little psychological ploys than at the dining table, the one place where parents, driven by their desperate need to feed, seem so ready to crumple and cave in? It's all good, healthy developmental stuff but extremely wearing, nevertheless, for the battle-weary souls who must cope with it.

☝ **Dr Sandi says:** 'No one likes to be powerless, to feel forced into something, even if it is for our 'own good'. Most humans have a need to empower themselves and that means making their own choices. So, a child's refusal to eat or to try new food may well be about trying to exert their own sense of self, their sense of who they are. Our self-identity is wrapped up in a whole range of issues, including what things we like. If others dictate what we must like, this can damage our sense of self which is so fragile at this age. And that's why gentle encouragement will win the day far more effectively than brute force.'

More practically, it's always worth bearing in mind that children often have erratic patterns of eating. It's not particularly unusual for them to have days where they eat little or nothing and then to fill up the next day.

> **Quite often, children are just too busy being children to bother with eating. Who wants to sit down and re-fuel when you can carry on playing?**

Another factor is that, by their very nature, children tend to be set in their ways. They like the safety and security of routine and, just as they like to know that a story follows their bath and that bed follows the story, they like to know what to expect at the supper table. Yet another reason why it can be hard sometimes to expand their dining horizons.

"Mine have their fits and fads, but don't all kids? At the moment my middle one will only eat vegetables raw and she won't eat meat at all. I've never been one to worry about food though, I go with the flow and am very laid back about it. I make no fuss, and offer no alternatives – they all end up eating okay and although my daughter may not be there quite yet, and I have to use a few tricks to get her to eat a good variety, I don't let it bother me. My eldest used to be fussy, too, but now, at seven, she'll eat anything I put in front of her. **"**

Sharron, mum to daughters aged seven, four and one

🍅 **Sally says:** 'Children these days are often too busy to be much bothered about their food. Their primary desire is to have fun, and to learn and develop through play. Free time to do this is often limited in the fast pace of the 21st century. This fast pace is often out of the child's hands and if, for instance, they're at school or nursery all day and then perhaps there are after-school activities, either theirs, or their siblings, then there is often little time for free play at home. Meals must sometimes seem like a waste of time in these situations.'

When older children are still being fussy

So, pre-schoolers are notoriously fussy and have lots of good reasons for it. But what about children who are older and, supposedly, wiser?

Although it's true to say that many children start to drop their fussy eating tendencies once they're at school full-time, plenty of kids are still giving their parents grief in the dining room well into the primary school years and beyond. This may be because their preferences have been so firmly established, old habits die hard. And they may still be subject to the same old attention-seeking and control-gaining ploys of toddlerdom. At this age, they're also more likely to be influenced by peer pressure and what they see in the media, so are more attracted to junk or 'fast' foods and, sadly, may even have concerns about body image or dieting that affect what they consume.

> **Regardless, the same rules apply when it comes to coaxing older kids to eat – almost all the suggestions in the next chapter are worth trying, whatever their age. (You may just find that older ones are wiser to your efforts than younger ones!)**

Dr Sandi says: 'Kids like to have easy explanations for things so if they eat something once and have an adverse reaction (which could be as benign as not liking it, or more severe – feeling sick, vomiting, or having a tummy ache, for example), they are quick to blame that food, even if the cause is completely unrelated.

So, catching a cold could be blamed on eating broccoli last night! This blame can be extrapolated to related food items – all green veg, or all meat, for example. It helps them assert some control in their world. They may also get fixed dislikes because they once had a mouthful that was too chewy, too hard, or too bitter. It's hard to get them to change these fixed views, as kids tend to think in black and white.'

Are they trying to tell me something?

Parents often fret that a refusal to eat is a sign that something's troubling their child. It might be, as any obvious change to their normal behaviour can indicate an emotional problem, so a sudden, or even gradual, reduction in appetite may set alarm bells ringing. (Similarly, a dramatic increase in appetite shouldn't be ignored – see chapter 4.)

> Watch out for major life events that could affect them – new baby, new house or new school are the most common ones. They could be using food as a means of getting your attention, so do keep an eye on their overall contentment with life.

Similarly, a simple comment made by some insensitive friend or relative ('My, you like your food don't you?', 'Look at her puppy fat', 'You're looking a little plump these days!' to give three examples) can set off a spiral of food aversion, too.

In this day and age, where body image can be an issue for children before they've even left primary school, the sad truth is that comments like these can be horribly significant.

Occasionally, a specific underlying psychological issue can cause a child to refuse food – for example, if they've developed a phobia of a specific food for some reason, perhaps caused by a bad choking experience. Other more general fears can also affect a child's inclination to eat, including fear of swallowing or vomiting. Such phobias are rare, and will more than likely require expert input to make right.

🍅 Dr Sandi says: 'I think parents will know when they have a serious psychological problem like this on their hands – for example, a child who only eats 'baby food' (for fear of choking) is clearly in need of professional help if they are still doing this by school age. The key point is whether or not their fears are adversely affecting them – for example, a fear of vomiting may be an issue but may not take over their life (they may just avoid certain food groups, for example). If their phobia limits their ability to live a normal life – if they won't go to parties, eat out, or eat at school, for example, then it's time to seek professional help.'

Psychological reasons why children act the way they do

★ **Dr Sandi says:** 'Knowing what makes kids behave the way they do is always useful – especially if you have some effective strategies up your sleeve to help you deal with that behaviour. This is particularly true when it comes to the business of eating. You may be reassured to know that most kids' reactions to your best attempts at keeping them healthy are perfectly normal, and there are good psychological reasons for them. Here are some insights into typical behavioural issues which are often linked to eating. Once you understand them, it's an awful lot easier to deal with them. Below we go though each issue and ways to deal with it.'

PSYCHOLOGICAL REACTANCE

The more something is forced upon us, the more we react against this assault on our freedom. We react, not just by refusing, but by adopting a contrary position. For example, try to stop them being friends with someone you disapprove of and the chances are that this particular friend will become all the more appealing. Similarly, if we try to force healthy food into our kids, they might react by deliberately seeking unhealthy options – this is known as psychological reactance, and it's not simply rebelling for the sake of it. It is an emotional reaction to having someone push their views on us and causes us (adults too) to adopt or strengthen opposing views.

Deal with it by:

Being laid-back about food issues. If you're aware of psychological reactance, you are more able to pre-empt it. Don't push the message too hard or you could have the opposite effect.

EMPOWERMENT AND CONTROL

We all need to feel empowered to make our own decisions and choices in life. Kids too, need to feel some empowerment and control. We live in a crazy, uncontrollable world in the main and this is even more true for kids who have very little control over the way their lives are run. They need some power over the clothes they wear, the activities they do, and yes, the food they eat. This is normal and to deny this basic human need is to ask for trouble.

Deal with it by:

Empowering your children to make their own healthy choices. Allow limited control and choice. So, take them to the supermarket and let them choose their own veg – the type and the actual selection of the produce; maybe they fancy prickly pear or starfruit? Maybe yellow pepper but not red? Coxes apples rather than Pink Lady? The point is that they will feel empowered rather than powerless. Let them choose what they have for pudding (from a limited range).

A NEED FOR ROUTINE

Kids need structure, routine and stability. They thrive on this. The world is uncertain, new and always changing for them – they cope best by knowing what is coming next and when. So, a good routine such as supper, bath, story time, cuddle, bed, helps them make the world safe and predictable. So too at mealtimes – they like to know what they are getting, that they will like it and that it is 'safe' (ie won't make them go 'yuck'). This is one reason why they are often reluctant to try new things.

Deal with it by:

Encouraging tastings without expecting them to eat the whole meal. For example, prepare their tried and trusted favourites but encourage them to start with a mouthful of something new. Knowing that they don't have to have the whole thing can feel safe and reassuring and they may be more open to new experiences this way.

A NEED TO REBEL OR TO BE INDEPENDENT

As kids grow, from toddlerdom they have a normal need to become independent of their parents, to become separate people with separate needs, attitudes and values. They may need to accentuate the differences between them and you in order to feel that they are sufficiently separate people. One way to do this is at the supper table, especially if you have made it clear that this is a very important issue for you. This is why some older children become vegetarian, vegan, or cheese-aversive, for example. It's a natural way of pointing out their growing independence from you.

Deal with it by:

Resisting the urge to quash rebellion. See it as a normal move towards independence and try not to take it as a personal affront on your culinary skills.

BLACK AND WHITE THINKING

Children tend to see the world as good or bad, black or white. Learning about shades of grey comes later in their development. This means that food is good or bad, tasty or not. And it can explain their stubbornness about trying new foods, or why they can be so resistant to food that they don't like the look of.

Deal with it by:

Teaching them gradually that things in general are rarely black or white. This is a gradual stage of development and not something that can be rushed. Look for opportunities (away from food) to get this message across; for example, show them that not everything is either brilliant or terrible – a film can be a bit good, or a day at school quite fun.

Medical or biochemical causes of fussy eating

Our child nutritionist, Sally, discusses possible reasons for fussy eating…

Sometimes, medical and biochemcial factors may be causing, or contributing to, a poor appetite or selective eating tendencies and it may be worth seeking to identify these so they can either be ruled out or tackled, before making the assumption that you've got a plain old fussy eater on your hands. It won't always be obvious which, if any, are relevant. If in doubt, your best bet is to consult a qualified nutritionist who can run tests and help to make appropriate changes to the diet.

ZINC DEFICIENCY

Insufficient levels of zinc (found in seafood, canned fish, lean red meat, green leafy vegetables, mushrooms, potatoes, nuts, seed, cereals, rice, rye, oats, lentils, pluses, wholegrains, cheese, wholemeal bread and eggs) can depress the appetite and affect tastes, creating preferences for strong or salty foods at the expense of a more balanced diet. If a diet is lacking in the zinc-rich foods mentioned above, a short course of supplementary zinc may help to redress the balance.

FOOD ALLERGY OR INTOLERANCES

Cravings for a particular food may, in a small number of cases, be a symptom of an allergy or intolerance to that food.

It may be worth seeking professional help in ruling out these potential causes for a child's selective eating.

BLOOD SUGAR IMBALANCE

Caused by a combination of too many refined foods which don't sustain energy, and low levels of the specific vitamins and minerals needed to regulate glucose in the body, fluctuating blood sugar levels can affect behaviour and appetite, which may create a 'fussy eater'. Blood sugar imbalance is easy to correct once identified by giving lots of small, regular meals and snacks; more slow-release carbohydrates like wholegrain bread and brown rice, and reducing sugar consumption.

CONSTIPATION

A 'bunged-up' child may well be disinclined to eat if their tummy feels full or uncomfortable. If they cannot easily open their bowels at least once a day they may need more fibre, which is best given in the form of fresh fruit and vegetables. (And even if they are 'regular', too much processed food can cause an accumulation of toxic matter in the bowel which can amount to a feeling of being constipated.) A course of friendly bacteria supplement (probiotics) may also help balance the gut.

ANAEMIA

A lack of available iron in the blood, which can cause poor appetite, nausea and fatigue. It's common in children who are fussy eaters (so there may well be a bit of a vicious circle in action) and caused by a lack of iron-rich foods such as lean red meat, fish, green leafy veg, wholegrains, fortified cereals, nuts, seeds, lentils, egg yolk, wheatgerm, wholemeal bread and dried fruits. If you can't convince them to eat more from this list of foods, supplements may be required to boost iron levels. (Iron works best with vitamin C, so it's good to try and serve iron-rich foods in conjunction with vitamin C-rich foods, so for example, boiled egg with orange juice, or broccoli with lentils are good combinations.)

LACK OF 'FRIENDLY' BACTERIA IN THE GUT

These affect appetite, digestion and bowel function. Levels can fall after a course of antibiotics or asthma medications, or during periods of stress. They can be boosted with a daily dose of live yoghurt or a short course of probiotics, which come in powder form from health food shops and can be sprinkled on food or in the guise of little yoghurt drinks (although these are usually high in sugar).

NAUSEA

This may be caused by zinc or iron deficiency, by a generally poor diet, or by anxiety and stress, and can affect the appetite. Again, supplements may help to redress the balance.

TOXIC METALS

Tiny traces of lead or aluminium which come from food, air, water and household products and sit in the body tissues are quite common and can deplete minerals. An excess can cause behavioural problems, which may make a child less than cooperative at the dining table.

Tiny tummies: respecting individual appetites

Many kids just don't have big appetites. It's perfectly normal – small children, after all, have small stomachs. And appetites vary a great deal throughout childhood in any case, according to activity levels and growth spurts.

Children's individual appetites need to be respected – indeed, it's important to encourage eaters of all sorts to be aware of their own appetite and not simply to guess or assume how hungry they are on any given day.

🍅 Sally says: 'Every individual has an individual appetite. Some people are always ravenous and others always eat tiny amounts. Who are we as parents to decide how hungry our children should be or how much food they require? Children's appetites are changeable. They can eat virtually nothing one day and then pig out the next. And they are likely to have different needs according to their age – and the size of their tummy.'

" I've recently learned that as kids we were always taught to eat everything on our plate, that waste is bad, and that we often pass that on to our own children, making mealtimes a battle which in turn can lead to rebellion and resentment. I now accept that if either of them says they are full then they probably are and I no longer try and force them to finish everything. We sometimes forget when we're loading their plates that their tummies are just not big enough for everything! "

Farzana, mum to kids aged eight and six

When exactly will they grow out it?

A child who is a fussy eater won't automatically become an adult fussy eater, especially if they've had the appropriate responses from people bringing them up. In fact, the vast majority of children drop their fussy eating tendencies as they get older.

> **Many start to eat a more varied diet after they go to school and become influenced – for the better – by what their peers are doing, and as they become generally more mature and open-minded about these things.**

Others get less selective as they go through their teens and reach early adulthood.

Some children continue to be fussy into their teens, and some never grow out of it. There are plenty of adults out there who are still very fussy indeed – but because they're adults, no-one really worries much about them. They may not be getting optimum levels of nutrition, but they're probably doing fine. (Although it must be said that experts are uncertain about the effects on long-term health.)

As a general rule though, fussy eating is something most children grow out of at some point on their journey to adulthood, as they develop the ability to make their own choices about food – and that's when being well informed about food will really come into play. If you want proof of this, just look around you. How many grown-ups do you know who require another person to pretend their food is a choo-choo train in order for them to eat it?

" My son was an extremely fussy eater as a pre-schooler for about four years. I can't really recall exactly when things started changing – I think it probably coincided with him starting school, but I do know that now he will eat almost everything I give him. I'm sure that for most of them it's just a phase they eventually grow out of. **"**

Suzi, mum to kids aged seven and five

◌ **Dr Sandi says:** 'It's worth considering that 'fussy eating' may not be such a big deal as we think – after all plenty of adults are fussy eaters to one degree or another, it's just that we notice it so much more in kids, and worry about it more. As adults, we make our own food and can pick or choose what we have according to our preferences, without anyone showing any concern for us. It's not the same for children, because they're not in charge.'

Is it time for a professional opinion?

A small number of children who have very severe or very long-term restricted eating habits may need some professional help to get them eating more, for the sake of their development and general health. This doesn't mean they have an 'eating disorder', just that they have a problem with food that needs addressing. It's a complex area, and it's impossible to say where perfectly normal childhood fussy eating ends and a problem requiring medical intervention begins: every child is different and every eating problem is considered different, too. As a general rule, if it's having an impact – whether physically, socially, or psychologically – on a child's life, then they should see a doctor.

While on the rise in lower age groups in recent years, full-blown eating disorders such as anorexia nervosa or bulimia nervosa are still extremely rare in children. They are very complex psychological conditions, and are by no means the automatic follow-on from any kind of fussy eating, although it's true that poor handling of fussy eating may be a contributory factor in any later development of an eating disorder, which is why it's so crucial when you have a fussy eater to stay cool about it.

Summary

- Fussy eating is a very common childhood tendency.

- Most kids go through it to one extent or another.

- There are many and varied reasons for fussy eating.

- Psychology plays a huge part, so how you deal with it is all-important.

- Pre-schoolers are most likely to be fussy eaters. But plenty of school-age children are picky, too.

- Understand their behaviour where food's concerned. It will help you deal with it.

- Occasionally, a child's refusal to eat can indicate an emotional problem. You may need to work out if anything else is troubling them.

- Physical, medical, or biochemical factors can sometimes be at play and it may be worth getting these ruled out by an expert.

- Fussy eating is by no means a prelude to eating disorders. But the wrong treatment of a fussy eater may be a factor in their development.

- Most kids simply grow out of fussy eating. It's a fact!

> - Fussy eating tendencies, even in the long term, will rarely be dangerous to health, but they can occasionally impact in a very serious way on a child's life. In these cases, it's time to seek help from your doctor.

References

1 Wardle and Cooke: Genetic and environmental determinants of children's food preferences, British Journal of Nutrition (2008).

5

Practical ways of dealing with difficult eaters

what this chapter covers:

- How to make a healthy diet the norm
- Be resilient
- Encourage open-mindedness
- Coping with conflict
- Make food look more appealing
- How to make unpopular foods popular
- Other children's eating habits
- Boosting their fruit and veg intake
- Don't forget to eat your own greens
- Make sure they're hungry
- If they refuse food, should I let them go hungry?

How to make a healthy diet the norm

The best way to help your kids eat a reasonably healthy, basically balanced diet, is to make it a simple matter of lifestyle for the whole family, and to lead the way in this yourself. If you do this from the start, it's a lot easier.

> **Even if you missed the boat on those early opportunities, it's never too late to start – you just need to do so with stealth and subtlety, so that no one really notices.**

Children pick up most of their behaviour cues from the influential adults around them, so if they see their parents eating healthily as a matter of course, they'll be far more likely to follow suit.

"I often find that when I pick up an apple and start eating it, one or both of my girls will pipe up, 'Can I have one?'**"**

Lorna, mum to daughters aged six and four

> **Graduated exposure techniques have been found by researchers to be helpful in encouraging fussy eaters to widen their diet[1], which suggests that if you keep on determinedly offering small amounts of a particular food to a child, there's a good chance that they'll come round to it eventually.**

Some healthy snack ideas

- Cup of unsalted home-popped popcorn

- Slice of fruit loaf

- Handful of dried fruit or nuts

- Fresh fruit smoothie

- Plain piece of sponge

- Warmed mini pitta

- Slice of wholemeal bread with margarine

- Slice of toast with humous or peanut butter

- Homemade flapjack

- Yoghurt

In fact, many children are actually quite prepared to try new foods, as long as they know they definitely have the option of disliking it. One reason why it's good to eat as a family is that it exposes them to the sights and smells of different foods on other people's plates (and allowing them to take a little from yours is an effective but subtle way to encourage them to sample stuff).

Eight ways to make healthy normal

1 Have a bowl of fruit permanently available, at their level. Let them know they can help themselves whenever they want (except just before a meal, when it might spoil their appetite).

2 Don't allow chocolate, sweets, cakes, crisps and other unhealthy foods to become 'everyday' foods, kept in the store cupboard as a matter of course. Just get them in at the weekend, or for special occasions only. And always have plenty of healthier alternative snacks and treats around so they never feel too hungry or hard done by, such as fruit, nuts, yoghurts, fresh wholemeal bread and butter, plain sponge cake, scones or flapjacks.

3 Encourage them to drink and enjoy water by serving it with every meal. Put it in a jug with some ice and have nice glasses or novelty beakers and straws to make it more appealing to little ones.

4 Make sure every meal comes with at least one sort of veg or salad accompaniment.

5 Even if you think you're a pretty healthy cook, chances are there are still areas you could reduce the levels of fat, sugar, and salt that the whole family is consuming. Make small, achievable changes to the way you cook and prepare food. If you do it in little bits, eventually it will become second nature.

6 Involve the kids in planning or preparing meals, snacks or menus. Ask them what they like and how to create a balanced and healthy meal out of their ideas. Most kids learn about 'five-a-day' and other basics about healthy eating in school, so build on this knowledge. Instead of healthy eating being imposed on them, they can feel part of the process.

7 Aim to make and serve healthy alternatives to their favourite 'junk' foods. For example, home-made burgers in wholemeal bread rolls, served with chunky oven chips and a 'side' of coleslaw, or homemade pizza with hidden veg in the topping.

8 Always offer them choices within a healthy range, so they feel in control without realising you're influencing what they eat.

Of course, it's entirely possible that a child has a perfectly genuine, inherent dislike for one or more specific foods and you will simply have to accept and respect that. Why shouldn't they? Most grown-ups have some disliked foods, after all – and you wouldn't tell an adult guest at a dinner party that they're not leaving the table until they've had at least three more mouthfuls of something they hate.

It's still worth taking a tenacious approach in the long-term, though, as children usually become more open-minded and less selective about food as they grow. Try coming back to it six months later.

"My daughter's infant school has introduced 'Try it Tuesday,' when parents are encouraged to put something new in their lunch boxes. I think it's a great idea – she's tried all sorts of things like mango, Edam, even chicken wraps instead of the usual Marmite sandwiches. It's an idea that might work well at home, too.**"**

Juliet, mum to kids aged nine, seven and four

Sally says: 'You need to persevere with offering new foods, but not excessively. Hence a theory that you try each food 10 times before giving up on it. It's just an average – beyond that, and you're probably flogging a dead horse. But that's not to say you couldn't try again some months or years down the line – after all, tastes change and taste buds get more sophisticated.'

Encourage open-mindedness

It's very easy to get stuck in a meal rut when you're feeding a family, particularly if one or more of your kids has a rather restrictive list of food preferences, or is just among those stubborn little people who know what they like and aren't much inclined to try anything new – after all, why bother preparing and serving something you know is going to end up in the bin?

> Children are more likely to be open-minded to new cuisine if they've been accustomed to different sorts of food from the start. But horizons can still be broadened later on in the game, if you do so with subtlety – introduce new things once in a while, and quietly and without fanfare.

Make a big deal out of trying new things and you're just asking for a negative reaction.

It may help to get them involved in creating new dishes. Or, take their favourite foods and try combining it in a different way, for example, if they like sausages, try dishing them up in the form of a sausage casserole, or a sausage and potato bake. You can squeeze extra veg into both for added nutrition and if you make sure the sausages are good quality with a high proportion of meat, you've got a healthy meal on your hands.

Be resilient

It's easy to become demoralised when kids won't eat the things you want and to just give in to their whims – you need to know that what you put in front of them has at least a fighting chance of being eaten. And quite apart from the overwhelming priority to get something – anything – down them, who needs the waste? It's not really surprising that a lot of families tend to have their menu choices set on a seven-day loop that never really changes.

But it is worth plugging away regardless; gently prompting them over and over again – without pressure – to try new things.

Coping with conflict

A fussy eater can strain parental tolerance to the utmost limits, but keeping cool is absolutely vital. If, as is often the case, they are refusing food to get attention or to seek control, then you'll be making things worse by reacting. So don't ever let them see that you're bothered. Easier said than done, it's true – there are few things more frustrating, particularly if you've spent time and effort on cooking. Try leaving the dining room for a few moments to cool down a little if you can really feel your temper rising. Ignore them, don't make a fuss, and don't get heavy. If it's clearly a no-go, quietly clear the table and leave it at that.

> Whatever you do, don't get cross. And never, ever force a
> child to eat something they don't want to.

Don't waste time picking up the under-fives on less significant stuff such as table manners, either – if you have a
seriously fussy eater on your hands, it's better for them to put
their food in their mouths with their fingers, for example,
than not to eat at all. If they're old enough to know better, try
not to nag about it – the aim is to make mealtimes happy
times and the dining room a happy place, and if they're
constantly being told off for not holding their cutlery right,
or sitting properly, they may start to develop negative
associations with sitting at the table.

> Be conscious, as ever, of the language you use.
> Always avoid 'labelling' a child as a fussy eater and
> actually using phrases like that in front of them (and even
> if you think you're having a private conversation with
> someone else about it, they could still be listening in). You
> may be subconsciously inviting them to live up to their
> reputation.

🍅 **Dr Sandi says:** 'There's no point making a
child eat something. They're likely to experience
'psychological reactance', which we all do when forced
to do something we don't want to. Basically, we rebel

and become determined to do the opposite. Forced to eat veg as a child? Most will rebel as an adult by eating more sweets! We really don't want to turn food into a battle of wills – we may win in the short-term but the long term losses might not be worth it.'

🍅 Sally says: 'Forcing it is counter-productive, and can lead to food aversion. Gentle persuasion and patience, however hard that may be, is the only way.'

HAVE A UNITED FRONT

A severe food refusing problem can cause a good deal of stress in the family, not least among parents who find themselves in disagreement about a way forward – quite possibly influenced by differing upbringings or childhood experiences of their own. Mums and dads need to have a united front though. You also need to get grandparents or any other influential adult who regularly feeds them, including childminders or nursery staff, on board. Avoid comparing their eating habits with that of brothers or sisters. Equally, it's important to be sensitive to the needs of the other children at your dining table, too.

Siblings who have to share a table with a seriously fussy eater can also be affected by the stress it causes, and may suffer from a lack of attention if their parents are focusing on the fussy eater. They may even develop referred eating problems – in order to try to wrest some attention they can use or abuse the situation to make things worse for their sibling, 'telling tales' on them for not eating their peas, for example, which is not a happy situation. So give equal attention to everyone who is at the table.

❝My husband was apparently very fussy when he was young, and our son Charlie seems to be the same. Mostly I'm prepared to be laid back about it, but I get very stressed when we eat with my mother-in-law, who will insist on hassling Charlie, telling him constantly to 'eat up' and even picking up his spoon to feed him sometimes.

My attitude is that if he doesn't like what I've given him, I just tell him calmly it's all there is, and if he wants to leave the table, I let him. I admit that when he hasn't eaten anything much for a day or two I can get very anxious, but then he'll suddenly eat loads, so I suppose he's getting everything he needs. Making faces or pictures out of food, and getting him to help with the preparation can be helpful, too.❞

Jane, mum to a son aged three

🍅 *Dr Sandi says*: 'Kids can become very confused by different messages. For example, one parent insists that they finish what's on their plate while the other lets them eat only what they want. I suggest parents sit down and thrash out an agreed philosophy, preferably with the aid of a book like this. Then you need to inform others, like grandma, who are regularly feeding them.'

How to make mealtimes as pleasant as possible

- Eat together as often as you can – it's a golden rule. In fact, even if you're not actually able to eat with them because your timetables are at odds, it's good to sit down with them, have a drink or a snack, and chat to them while they eat.

- Allow them a degree of autonomy and control at mealtimes – let little ones feed and serve themselves as soon as they're able and allow older children to make a selection from a couple of options, wherever possible.

- Don't give them too much choice, though – they may start to expect it, it's more work for you and inevitably, there'll be more waste.

- Distraction can help. Taking their mind off what they're eating – or rather, what they're not eating – is a time-honoured tradition among desperate parents who'll do anything to see their kids' dinner go down.

- As a general rule, if you have a fairly serious case of food refusal on your hands, then anything goes – some parents allow their children to have favourite games or toys at the table, sing songs, read to them, or indulge in complex role play of some sort of other. If this really works, then go ahead, but if not, ditch it quick. And don't let it become a permanent habit, if you don't want to have to keep doing it permanently.

- Be relaxed and don't rush mealtimes. Equally, don't allow them to become too drawn out, especially if you've reached a deadlock. If you haven't got them to eat as much as you'd like to within half an hour, give up and calmly clear the table. Don't immediately scrape their rejected food into the bin, though. If they claim to be hungry later on, you can always offer to re-heat it for them.

A CHANGE OF SCENERY CAN CAUSE A CHANGE OF HEART

Although set mealtimes and eating at the table are more likely in the long run to encourage healthy eating habits, there's no point insisting on them if mealtimes have become routinely miserable. Getting any kind of good food down them will be your priority, and if you're struggling to do that then it's perfectly okay to let the other stuff slide for a while. It's fine to let them 'graze' very occasionally if that's what it takes – children are often inclined towards this way of eating anyway, and can be fazed by large platefuls of food. Offer a wide variety of nutritious morsels, wherever possible: chopped fruit and veg, nuts and seeds, small sandwiches, cubes of cheese. 'Picnicking' in this way can be a great way of getting food down your child, but shouldn't replace proper meals on a permanent basis – your aim should still be for the norm to be to sit at the table.

> A little attention to geography can sometimes lift the pressure caused by a succession of miserable mealtimes. You may find you can get a good (or at least, a reasonable) amount down them simply by eating in the garden, visiting a local restaurant, setting up a teddy bears' picnic in the lounge, or having tea at a friend's.

Some parents find that if they let them eat while watching their favourite television programme, their children will put food into their mouths without really thinking about it. The odd TV dinner here and there – no more than once weekly, say – is fine for a special treat. But they really do need to be carefully rationed because if you allow it to become habitual you might not get them back to the table, which is the only place they're going to truly learn to be happy, healthy eaters. If you do allow TV dinners once in a while, put them in the room with the television in – don't be tempted to bring the box into the dining room. And make it clear that if they ever become too distracted to eat, that this particular treat will cease.

Make food look more appealing

The right presentation can help foods seem more appealing to children, especially toddlers who are sometimes impressed by these things. Small children tend to favour dainty looking portions (indeed, it's often all they can stomach, anyway), and may balk if different foods on a plate are mixed, so serve the different components of the meal separately if they so desire. Don't try sneaking something they don't like on a plate of something they do – chances are, they'll reject both.

> **If you've got the time and energy to fashion food into clown faces and treasure islands, then feel free, but don't make a rod for your own back by having to get creative every time in order for them to contemplate eating something.**

That said, you may well find that a little attention to detail can make a huge difference. For instance, you can make sandwiches or slices of fruit or vegetables into flowers or stars fairly easily with the aid of a biscuit cutter, or make fish cakes fish-shaped without any great creative talent required.

You could also allow them to 'play' with their food sometimes – although traditionally this is considered bad manners, needs must, and if the opportunity to shape a funny face out of their lunch or painstakingly thread peas on to a kebab skewer has the useful side effect of them actually eating it afterwards, then so be it.

" The smallest effort in presentation can make a difference when it comes to getting my daughter to eat. For instance, she used to refuse to eat mashed potato until I started serving it in neat, round balls made with an ice cream scoop. She won't eat massive chunks of cheese, but when I grate it, or cut it into tiny little cubes, that's fine. There are limits of course – I'm not prepared to stand in the kitchen all day carving flowers out of carrots and creating elaborate pictures with the food on her plate. But I am happy to put in a bit of effort if it means the difference between her eating and not eating. "

Lorna, mum to daughters aged six and four

" I found that making pancakes and serving them with a bunch of fruit and veg so he can make faces on them was popular. I also invented the 'peabab' for him – skewering peas onto a cocktail stick. It's a bit of an effort, but it's worth it. **"**

Joanne, mum to kids aged eight and five

"Although she loathes milk and almost all varieties of cheese, my daughter will eat Babybel and yoghurt, so I know she's probably getting all the calcium she needs from those. My other one claims she hates 'all veg', but actually she will eat broccoli and peas. I reckon that if you search hard enough, there'll usually be something that they like from each food group. **"**

Deborah, mum to kids aged seven, five, and two

Other children's eating habits

Other children can be influential, for better or worse. Invite all the good eaters you know to tea regularly to set a good example – but don't bang on about them being better eaters than yours, which could frankly be hurtful and certainly won't be productive. If an even fussier friend is coming over, offer something you know is tried and tested by both of them, served up in a fun way, picnic style, perhaps.

Ignore other parents who are smug about the fact that their kids will eat anything, or make negative comments about your child's habits. If you let this kind of attitude get to you, it may cause tension and guilt which certainly won't help matters. Reassure yourself with the knowledge that fussy eating is very common, and very normal.

How to make unpopular foods popular

Try thinking laterally if your child refuses point blank to eat a certain food that you know they need.

For instance, loads of kids won't eat fish when it's dished up on a plate as it is, but few will turn it down if it's coated in breadcrumbs to create fish fingers or blended with potato to make fish cakes. (Made with half wholemeal/half white breadcrumbs, and oven baked, or shallow fried in olive oil, these are healthy, as well as popular offerings, especially if you use fresh tuna, mackerel, or salmon, for a healthy dose of Omega 3.*) Other ideas for simple, healthy fish dishes they might try are kedgeree or sardines on toast. And if fish is a still a complete no-no, you can always sneak in some essential fatty acids by grinding nuts and seeds onto salads, cereals, or fruit crumble toppings; or in the form of oils added to salad dressings, cooked vegetables, rice or pasta.

Build on the foods they do like. If they're big on bread, explore all the different sorts as a way of opening their eyes to new tastes: try pittas, tortillas, or seedy batches and look at different ways you could dish it up with added nutritional value – coating a slice of bread in beaten egg and frying it to make French toast, for example, will boost its protein value.

(* Canned tuna, although still a nutritious option, doesn't count as an oily fish because most of the healthy fats are lost during the canning process. However, other canned fish still count as oily fish.)

"When he was a baby I gave my son as wide a variety of food as I could, but around 13 months he learnt that he could say no and started to refuse more and more food. He's now four and has a range of about 20 foods he will eat (I know because I've written them all down). He won't even eat fairly basic stuff that most children like such as pasta, eggs, potatoes, pizza, baked beans. I've tried every technique in the book to get him to try new foods, and now my basic policy is to ensure that what he does get is good quality. I bake all our bread, so on the days when he will only eat toast, at least I know it's decent stuff. I also give both my kids a multi-vitamin every day. I try not to stress about it, but it's very hard, and it gets me down sometimes. The worst is when you try to explain it to other people. He's recently started school, so I've been inviting his friends round but tend to avoid the return invites because I can't bear having to explain the food situation to other mums. I hate to think of him being judged for it. Ultimately I take solace in the fact that he's generally a healthy child with lots of energy who sleeps well, so somewhere along the line he must be getting enough nutrition."

Joanne, mum to kids aged eight and five

Boosting their fruit and veg intake

Children are notoriously pernickity about fruit and vegetables – in fact, research shows that it's a pretty much universal tendency[2] and that kids simply have an innate preference for sweet, starchy and high fat foods over fruit, veg and protein.[3] There may be more specific reasons for it, too – one study has found that some children's genetic code makes them particularly sensitive to a bitter tasting chemical found in vegetables[4].

If you do have a fruit 'n' vegavoider on your hands, try not to panic. Few children won't eat any at all, and while a good mix of different varieties, colours and nutrients is the ideal, they can do pretty well on just a handful.

> **You may be reassured to know that for children, a surprisingly small quantity of fruit or vegetables counts as one of their recommended five-a-day portions – see the chart on page 12 for more information.**

There are many and varied ways in which you can get fruit and veg into fussy eaters without them necessarily realising it, for example:

- Blending them into sauces, soups and stews

- Sprinkling them finely chopped over pizzas or cereals

- Serving up delicious smoothies

One word of warning: don't lie outright about what's in their food. If they rumble you and discover those finely chopped mushrooms, or detect the presence of pulped courgettes with their finely honed detector senses, they could end up suspicious of everything you later put in front of them.

In general, it's much better if you can get them to appreciate fruit and vegetables (indeed, all nutritious foods) as something to be appreciated and enjoyed for what they are. And the best way to do that is to be upfront about it.

🍅 **Sally says:** 'In the interests of their health, stealth is sometimes needed. Children cannot take responsibility for their own wellbeing when they're young. That's our job, and I believe that 'hiding' good foods is sometimes justified.'

🍅 **Dr Sandi says:** 'There's nothing wrong with the fine art of getting healthy stuff in without them realising. But I'm against sneaking hated foods into dishes and then pretending you haven't, which I think is a different thing. For example, if your child loathes cheese and you make a dish that requires cheese, I don't think it is good to pretend you didn't put cheese in, either lying by omission or outright to their query. I think this can lead to mistrust and this could be far more dangerous than them missing out on a food group.'

BE RESILIENT WHEN IT COMES TO OFFERING FRUIT AND VEGETABLES

Gillian Harris's research[5] found that babies tend to 'categorise' food by colour, so if they try something green and don't like it, that may lead them to reject other green foods before they've even tried them.

So, if they reject one type of fruit or veg, give them an alternative and remember to try again with it a bit later. And keep on serving up all sorts of different colours to get them used to the idea that food comes in an array of shades.

🍅 Sally says: 'Brightly coloured, natural, fresh foods are rich in the vital antioxidants needed for health and wellbeing – and fortunately they often look appealing, too.'

DON'T FORGET TO EAT YOUR OWN GREENS

Check your own eating habits before fretting too much over theirs. As we've already pointed out, kids learn direct from their nearest and dearest – in fact, research has shown that very young children are more likely to eat when they see other people sitting near them are eating[6], which is another reason why it's beneficial to eat as a family whenever you can.

> If you turn your nose up at vegetables, eat restrictively, or
> make a big fuss about certain foods, then you can't really
> expect anything better from your children.

If you must be a fussy eater, try and be one without them
realising.

Make sure they're hungry

One fairly obvious reason kids don't eat much at dinner is
that they've been filling up beforehand. The simple solution
is to stop them snacking too much and at the wrong times.
Of course, you need to bear in mind that kids of all ages will
usually need some snacks to keep their energy and blood
sugar levels on an even keel, but as a general rule, don't give
them anything – with the exception perhaps of fruit or
vegetables – for an hour before meals, and when you do give
them snacks, stick to small portions of something nutritious
like fruit and veg, yoghurts, cheese, or something carb-based
such as bread, scone or plain sponge.

Be aware that fluids can fill them up too, particularly milk or
fizzy drinks. While a good source of useful nutrients and
protein, milk (including milk-based foods) should be limited
to no more than a pint a day. And fizzy drinks provide
nothing in the way of nutrition, anyway, so are best avoided
altogether.

How to make fruit and vegetables more appealing

- Try offering 'baby' versions of fruit and veg which are less intimidating – cherry tomatoes and miniature sweetcorn, for example.

- Don't overcook veg as they're horrible when soggy. Stir frying is a good way to cook lightly. If they don't like them cooked at all, just give them raw instead. A dip served in a small bowl can add appeal.

- Freeze grapes – they turn into cute little fruit lollies.

- Give veg just before a main course, as an appetiser, rather than with it. If they're really hungry, they're more likely to indulge.

- Make a fruit salad, with the fruit peeled and sliced in a little fruit juice, perhaps served with a dollop of ice cream.

- Quietly place small dishes of sliced or diced raw veg next to them when they're engaged in some other activity.

- They may dig in without even thinking about it. Plates with compartments with different items offered separately are often appealing.

- Serve peas and carrots buttered, or strawberries and bananas with a chocolate dip. (Not all the time, mind...)

- Aim to serve up veg as fresh as possible and while it's in season – the flavour's always 10 times better.

- Pick your own where possible. Peas still in the pod are great fun to pop – and completely irresistible!

- Call them something different. Broccoli becomes 'trees' for example (and children who eat them are therefore 'giraffes') and peas become 'mini footballs'.

- Offer fruit and raw veg sliced, diced, segmented or cut into dainty juliennes. (And, although much of the goodness is in the skin, peeled if they insist.)

- Try roasting veg. It gives a lovely sweet flavour.

- Try stewing fruit. Sometimes kids prefer a softer texture. Add ice cream or crumble to enhance enjoyment.

It can help to have a good routine for mealtimes and snacks, so they know what they can expect and when. And make sure you're the person dishing snacks out – don't get into the habit of allowing them to plunder the store cupboards whenever the fancy takes them.

> **“**If my son has anything more than an apple mid-afternoon, then he won't really eat his tea. I fell into a major snack trap with his older sister when she was two or three, with the result that she lived on biscuits and raisins, and barely ate her main meals.**”**
>
> *Juliet, mum to kids aged nine, seven and four*

If they refuse food, should I let them go hungry?

Don't pander to your fussy eater by creating meals specially for them. Your aim should be to offer one meal at each sitting, and to make sure they know that's their only option because if they know there is always another possibility on the menu, or the chance of a tasty snack later on instead, they'll have little incentive to try what you give them at first. And anyway, who needs the extra work? Of course, no-one likes the idea of sending their children to bed hungry. The way round it is to always make sure there's at least one fairly nutritious component of the meal that you know they will eat, and that way, you know they will at least have had something.

> You shouldn't give in to demands for any old junk in these circumstances, even if you feel that anything would be better than nothing.

Frankly, if what they're eating is of no nutritional value at all, they really might as well go hungry.

Avoid using bribery

It's tempting when you've got a fussy eater on your hands to use any method of persuasion open to you to get food down them.

> But however desperate you get, don't be tempted to offer one sort of food as bribery or reward in order to get another sort inside them – telling them they can have chocolate afterwards if they eat their greens, for example.

It puts an inflated value on the chocolate and it doesn't do much for their associations with the greens, either, as it makes them into a mere stumbling block to be tolerated in order to get to the grand prize. Chocolate, crisps, biscuits and other treats are all fine when given in moderate quantities as part of a balanced diet, but they shouldn't be linked to a fussy eater's acceptance of other less 'desirable' foods. It is, however, perfectly reasonable to say to a child that they need to finish or at least make a good attempt at their main course before having their pudding, on the basis that pudding only ever comes after a reasonable amount of dinner's been consumed.

> Most experts are dubious about the use of rewards of any kind in connection with eating habits. That's because if you make a big deal out of what they do and don't eat, they'll quickly come to realise how important it is to you – and may well choose to use that to their psychological advantage.

Also, they may come to expect to be rewarded every time, when in fact you want them to see it as ordinary behaviour. So, while it's natural to want to offer some kind of reward or to heap lavish praise on a problematically fussy eater who's tried something new, made a good effort, or got down something they claimed previously to dislike, it's better to be quietly positive about it than to big it up as some great achievement.

🍅 **Dr Sandi says:** 'Generally speaking, bribery isn't to be encouraged but I do think it's advisable not to allow 'afters' until your children have at least tried a meal, or had at least a few mouthfuls of their veg – not bribery as such, but on the basis that if they are too full for their veg then they must be too full for afters, too.

Nor is it a good idea to give 'rewards' for clean plates, because this can encourage eating for the wrong reasons – purely to earn the rewards, or to please a parent, for example, and this can lead to an association of pleasing people with food consumption which is not a healthy link.

However, I do think that adding a sticker to a chart for every portion of their five-a-day fruit and vegetables is a good idea – not by way of reward necessarily, but simply to help them chart their progress in making this goal. Children usually like this kind of activity so it puts a really positive spin on their five-a-day efforts.'

What children need to survive

Some children take food refusal to such an extreme that it becomes a huge worry for parents, who may wonder how they can actually survive on such small quantities, or such a limited menu. The reassuring truth is that, in the majority of cases, even fairly extreme food refusers will be doing okay.

> If you're worried that your child isn't getting enough nutritionally, sit down and write a list of every little thing they've eaten or drunk over the course of the week. You may find it's a bigger or more diverse list than you realised – or, at the very least, that it is quite enough to keep them alive.

Even if what they eat seems limited, chances are there'll be something from each major food group that they will eat. That's why, if you've got a fussy eater, it's useful to have a rough grasp of what the groups are, what's in them, and what they do for us. If they won't touch milk, for example, they may be able to get the important nutrients (it provides calcium, essential for healthy bones and teeth; and vitamins K, A, B2, and D, which is needed to absorb calcium) from other dairy products such as cheese or yoghurt, or from alternative sources such as broccoli, canned salmon, and nuts.

Problems are most likely to arise if they're missing out on one or more entire food groups, so the child who will only eat jam sandwiches and never lets a piece of fruit or veg pass their lips may be seriously deficient in vital specific nutrients such as vitamin C or fibre. It's possible to get by even on a very restrictive diet like this for quite long periods of time – and many children do, often without any obvious health problems as a result (as many a dining room conflict veteran will tell you.) But clearly, these kind of eaters will not be enjoying optimum health. If you've tried everything and you really are concerned about a major lack of something or other, then you may want to consider a supplement.

> **If it's a problem that's being ongoing for more than a couple of months, then you should probably seek some medical or nutritional advice.**

🍅 **Sally says:** 'Nutrients are best taken from food sources, but for fussy eaters who just aren't getting a balanced diet, a specific multi-vitamin suited to their age may help to reassure a worried parent that at least the recommended daily amount of vitamins and minerals is going in. And if a specific vitamin or mineral is suspected or proven to be deficient in a child – such as calcium, iron or zinc for instance – and that in turn may be exacerbating the problem because a lack of these things can suppress the appetitie and affect tastes, then a supplement is certainly a good idea, to allow the body to rebalance itself.

Essential fatty acids, which recent research has shown may be linked to learning and behaviour, can also be supplemented, which is useful, since many children simply don't like the foods which contain EFAs, such as oily fish, nuts, seeds and green veg.

Supplements do not, however, replace all the benefits found in foods, for example fibre, protein and specific plant nutrients which cannot be replicated. So they can't be relied upon as replacements for food in the long-term.'

❝My son Ben was never a good eater. As a small child he lived on bacon, crisps, meat and bread, and very little else – fruit and veg never passed his lips. He continued like that for many years, and eventually I gave up trying. Somewhere along the way he began to eat fairly normally and he's now a strapping 25-year-old with no apparent health problems – so far."

Pat, mother to son

"I have two children and have placed great importance on feeding them, to the point that the success I feel as a mother seems to be directly proportionate to my ability to providing them with a healthy and nourishing diet. This was all well and good with my first, who went through the weaning stage with no issues. He gratefully ate every mouthful of carefully prepared organic produce I put in front of him and I felt like a Supermum. Then came my daughter, who rejected most foods and, of course, I had much less time to concentrate on her. As a result I felt a complete failure and was in a state of constant panic about the lack of nourishment she was receiving. Although two years on I am slightly more relaxed, she still eats very little for my liking and only ever eats one meal a day – sometimes breakfast, sometimes lunch and occasionally tea.

Perhaps I am being too obsessive, but I still worry that she's missing out on nutrients. After speaking with the doctor, I'm now giving her a daily dose of multi-vitamin syrup."

Ginny, mum to kids aged three and two

⊘ Sally says: 'Fussy eaters are a relatively modern phenomenon – they didn't really exist before the advent of mass food manufacturing and processing, when food was scarce and eaten as a family, mothers were full-time mums, and discipline was stricter. It may even be that the deficiencies of the modern diet that have caused the fussy eating, rather than the other way round. The truth is, we cannot be sure if long-term fussy eating can cause damage to health.'

What to do if you're still worried...

If you're concerned that your child's growth or general health is being affected by their dodgy eating habits in any way – for instance because their energy levels seem low, they have poor concentration, they have rotten immunity and always seem to have colds or infections, or their pallor is unusual – you should make an appointment with your GP. Don't hesitate to seek help, too, if you suspect they have a serious emotional issue linked to their eating. If necessary, you should get a referral to an appropriate expert, whether that be a nutritionist, dietitian, psychiatrist or specialist paediatrician.

Summary

- Resilience is essential – you need to keep on trying to widen their horizons, however frustrating the waste may be.

- If they won't eat a particular food, try serving it differently.

- Experiment with the foods they do like.

- Don't let them see how much it means to you.

- If they won't eat, never force them.

- Don't label a child a 'fussy eater' – and avoid comparing them with others.

- Make sure you, your partner and any other adults who feed them regularly share a common strategy for dealing with the problem.

- Try something different to encourage appetites – such as a picnic, or a meal out.

- Presentation counts for a lot. Don't go overboard, but it's worth putting some thought into the way you dish things up.

- If you're worried that they're not eating enough, try jotting down everything they eat and drink in a week. You may be surprised to find it's more than you thought.

- Don't offer them a whole new dinner if they rejected what you offered.

- Don't 'bribe' them to eat, particularly not with other types of food.

- A wide variety of fruit and veg is ideal – but some is definitely better than nothing.

- Set the right example. If your eating habits are bad you can't expect theirs not to be.

- Make sure they're hungry! Keep snacks light and avoid them just before dinner. Watch for filling drinks, too.

References

1 Wardle et al: Increasing children's acceptance of vegetables, a randomised trial of parent-led exposure (2003).

2 Cooke et al: Demographic, familial and trait predictors of fruit and vegetable consumption by pre-school children, Public Health Nutrition (2004).

3 Wardle et al: Factor-analytic structure of food preferences in four-year-old children in the UK, Appetite (2001).

4 Bell and Tepper: Short-term vegetable intake by young children classified by 6-n-propylthoiuracil bitter-taste phenotype, American Journal of Clinical Nutrition (2006).

5 Greville-Harris: Towards an understanding of how young children make and overcome neophobic food responses (2004).

6 Harper and Sanders: The effect of adults' eating on young children's acceptance of unfamiliar foods, Journal of Experimental Child Psychology (1975).

6

Dealing with 'food junkies'

what this chapter covers:

- You don't have to be overweight to be unhealthy
- Cut out unhealthy snacks
- What they're eating when they're not with you
- Swapping bad habits for good
- Making sure they have enough to eat
- Keep a limit on choices
- Setting the right example: Why it's *still* the most important thing you can do!
- Why it's *still* okay to indulge sometimes

You don't have to be overweight to be unhealthy

A child doesn't necessarily need to be overweight to be in possession of very unhealthy eating habits – fact is, some kids are less prone to gaining weight than others, just like adults. But although slim children who eat too much 'junk' food may not be as obviously at risk of health problems as chubbier ones, that doesn't mean they're not potentially storing them up.

Too much junk is thought to cause or contribute to a whole range of health problems in kids such as tiredness, poor concentration, lack of energy, mood swings, bowel problems, tummy aches, headaches and nausea, frequent colds and other infections. An overload of salt, hydrogenated fats, sugars, additives and processed, low-fibre foods can all affect blood sugar levels and digestion for the worst. And there's all sorts of evidence that junk food isn't a good influence on behaviour, and that it can even affect brain power.

> **One survey, for example, found that children who regularly eat junk food are nearly three times more likely to behave badly than those who avoid it, and that SATS scores are 11% higher in kids eating a good diet than those eating a poor one[1].**

Besides all that, ditching childhood junk habits is about far more than just keeping an eye on their weight – it's about setting up healthy eating habits that will stand them in good stead for life. All of which is far easier said than done. Junk food is hard – in fact, impossible – to avoid these days. It's everywhere, and it's big business too, which means that even if you did strive to keep it out of your own home, they'd be exposed to it from many other sources. And the chemicals found in some processed foods can actually be both physically and psychologically addictive, so the more they have, the more they may crave.

> **If your children already have a predilection for junk, you may have a tough task on your hands helping them to cut down. But it can be done. The trick is to make a subtle overhaul of the whole family's lifestyle habits.**

🍅 **Sally says:** 'If you're trying to change entrenched habits, it will take a little while and you will need to be patient and have nerves of steel to stick to your goal. Be firm and consistent, but be flexible. There'll be times when you feel like you are taking three steps forward and two steps back, but bear with it; they'll get used to it in the end.'

Cut out unhealthy snacks

You may find that cutting out any high-sugar, high-fat snacks and drinks that are consumed in between meals is all you need to do to address a child's junk food problem. Be cautious about cutting back on snacks completely, though. Children should never be refused between-meal sustenance when they need it (and generally speaking that will be once midmorning and once in the afternoon, particularly after school), as their blood sugar levels will dip and they'll simply be ravenous by the time they are served a meal and then likely to gorge themselves: just make sure the snack you give them is a healthy one (see the table below for some suggestions).

Don't refuse them a bedtime snack either, as these are important in maintaining blood sugar levels in the night and improve the quality of their sleep – just make sure it's light, nutritious, and easily digested – for example, yoghurt or a bowl of non-sugary cereal. If they're still complaining, serve up some other distraction instead, like an extra bedtime story.

> If they seem really hungry after school and a small healthy snack doesn't seem to help much, you may have to consider an earlier tea-time – although ideally this will still involve the whole family.

Some unhealthy/healthy snack swaps

SWAP...	FOR...
a bag of crisps	a bowl of unsalted home-popped popcorn
a bar of chocolate	a slice of fruit loaf
sweeties	a handful of dried fruit or nuts
a can of cola	a fresh fruit smoothie
a chocolate biscuit	a plain piece of sponge
a slice of chocolate cake	a warmed mini pitta
a toasted cheese sandwich	a slice of toast with humous or peanut butter
a bowl of ice cream	a yoghurt

What they're eating when they're not with you

Schools these days are coming round – thank you, Jamie Oliver – to the notion of healthier eating, and your kid's school canteen may not be the turkey twizzling minefield it once was. In fact the government recently issued a whole series of plans to improve school catering services across the board which have already begun with the banning of sales of confectionery and other unhealthy snacks. And all school

Packing it in... some lunchbox ideas

- Pitta breads stuffed with humous and salad

- Wraps filled with cold meat, pickle or mild mustard, and cherry tomatoes

- Bagel with cream cheese and cucumber or turkey and pickle

- Container of tuna blended with half yoghurt and half mayo, served with crispbreads

- Tub of prawns in coleslaw

- Mini sausages served with a small pot of ketchup

- Cherry tomatoes and cubes of cheese

- Tea loaf, muesli slice or mini banana muffin

- Tortilla chips, pretzels or vegetable crisps rather than crisps

- Fruit crisps

- Popcorn

- Fruit such as a handful of grapes, a peeled satsuma or a small banana lunches (as of September 2009) will have to meet certain nutritional standards. Which is just as well, because what they eat when they are at school constitutes a fairly significant part of their diet. Meanwhile, schools generally display a menu, so you can check out what's on offer, and if you're not sure what exactly is in school meals or how they are made, ask to speak to the cook and find out for yourself.

If you give them a packed lunch, there are some simple guidelines to ensure that what goes in will constitute a reasonably balanced meal. Include:

- **A starchy carb-based food such as bread or rice**

- **Some protein in the form of fish, meat, eggs, cheese or nuts**

- **A dairy food for calcium such as milk, cheese or yoghurt**

- **At least one portion of fruit and/or veg – peel and slice or chop to make them more appetising**

- **A drink of water, milk or diluted fruit juice.**

- **If you include a 'treat' food try and stick to plain popcorn, a homemade flapjack or a piece of plain sponge.**

❝Peer pressure really kicks in at school lunchtime. I've had grief from my six-year-old already – one friend has a chocolate biscuit every day in their lunch box and another has a sausage roll and a doughnut! What on earth are you supposed to say about that? Persistence does pay off, though, because she seems to have stopped complaining lately. I can't bear to think of her being disappointed when she opens it, though, so I stick in a small 'treat' on most days. It's usually a healthy(ish) version – a piece of homemade cake, some no-salt crisps, or plain popcorn, and she seems happy with that."

Lorna, mum to daughters aged six and four

☺ **Sally says:** 'Recent media coverage has highlighted that packed lunches can be worse than school meals. However, although there is obviously a need to clean them up, one needs to be mindful of peer group pressure. It's excruciatingly embarrassing to be chomping through sprouted seeds when your mates are eating sausage rolls. This is the territory for the '75% rule' – feed them well at home and relax a little on the lunch box while maintaining sensible nutritional standards.

Anyway, if you insist on giving them brown bread when they only like white, they'll just swap it or chuck it away. There's no point at all in persisting in including food you know they don't like. There's a story about the banana that knew its own way home eventually, as the recipient's mother had put it back in the lunch box every day for a week. I would give up at that stage, and try grapes instead.'

🍎 **Dr Sandi says:** 'With packed lunches, there's the added psychological pressure on mums to provide treats – not just for peer pressure reasons, but also to send a message to your child in your absence that you love them when you are not there to show it personally. We imagine their delight at seeing their treat and imagine them basking in our love. Conversely, an unappetising lunch might leave them feeling unloved – 'mum doesn't love me enough to bother about making me happy'. So, the psychological pressure to make their packed lunch an enjoyable experience is immense. The answer? It has to lie in providing 'healthy' treats like homemade popcorn and flapjacks. You could also put some other non-edible treats in occasionally to 'show' your love – stickers or football cards, for example.'

Whether they have a school lunch or a packed lunch, the fact is you still can't influence exactly what they eat when they're not with you. That's true even if you give them a carefully packed lunch – they can after all just leave whatever they don't want, and on many a packed lunch table, an active 'swapsie' system exists which means that goodies from other children's lunch boxes will find their way into yours.

A certain amount of 'letting go' is called for when it comes to what our kids consume outside of the home. As parents, we have to accept that once they are out of eyeshot we can't control everything they put in their mouths.

But they'll be okay as long as they eat well most of the time. Try and foster honesty so you at least have an idea what they've been eating and when. One way to do this is to be very relaxed when they do tell you what they've eaten. If they know there are foods available that fill you with horror at the thought of them eating, then that might just make them more appealing.

🍅 **Sally says:** 'Moderation is the key. They'll get hold of the junk without you so all you can do is make sure the home diet is healthy and accept the rest as part of life. Instilling good habits in children usually pays off when they're adults even if they do deviate for a while once they're old enough to choose – that's all part of growing up, and pushing the boundaries. But don't make too big a deal out of it – you don't want to pass on unhealthy obsessions with healthy eating.'

🍅 **Dr Sandi says:** 'Parents can drive themselves mad worrying about every little thing that their kids eat. They should look at the overall picture and in the context of their general lifestyle. I certainly think that if a child is very active then a small 'treat' at lunch and even one after school is not likely to harm them.

Kids with more sedentary lifestyles may need more care in terms of their diets – and isn't this true of adults, too? It's really about taking a holistic approach to their lifestyles, rather than worrying about every little chocolate biscuit that goes into their lunch box.'

Swapping bad habits for good

Overhauling well-established habits is never going to be easy, but it's something you'll need to do if you're concerned about a child's junk food consumption. If treats and sweets are something you've got into the habit of doling out daily, aim to wean them off such a regular intake. They shouldn't feel deprived just because a day has gone by when they haven't had a 'goodie' of some sort.

> **The easiest way to cut down on sweets, crisps and other treat foods is not to put them in your shopping trolley or to have them in the house as a matter of routine – if they're not in the cupboard, they can't have them.**

If you do have them at home, keep them somewhere inaccessible to them and dole them out at your own discretion. And make sure you have lots of healthier snacks available as alternatives – they'll stop complaining eventually.

Look out for food associations that may have become ingrained in your family's life and think about ways that you can break the pattern. One classic example is the TV snack: have your kids come to associate the telly being switched on at a particular time of day with the ceremonial opening of a bag of crisps, for example? Snacking while watching telly isn't great, anyway, as it can lead to what's called unconscious eating – in other words, shovelling food in without much consideration as to whether it's needed or not. One simple way to avoid after-school snacking in front of the television is to take them something to eat on the way home from school, instead.

> **If you want to change a family habit, aim to do so with subtlety if you want to avoid being unpopular.**

Don't make a dramatic announcement that things are about to change and aim to use the most positive language you can when trying to 'sell' a new habit to children. So, for instance, rather than forcing the point that crisps and pop are from now subject to rationing, emphasise that you're all going to try and up the amount of fruit and water you consume. If you can justify lifestyle changes without even mentioning health or weight, then by all means do so: for instance, maybe you want to ban snacking upstairs because you're launching a keep-the-place-tidy drive, or you're all going to start eating more exotic fruit in the pursuit of experimentation. It may be a little easier for them to accept that sort of reasoning without feeling deprived.

> **Don't forget that habits can be a useful thing, too. Once children (and it works for adults, too) become used to certain food habits or associations, they won't even think about asking for something different – eventually.**

"I remember always being given biscuits, a bit of cake or some crisps after school while sitting in front of the telly. It was always a lovely way to chill out after school. To this day I still associate television with eating. I still have to eat something sweet or salty while watching telly in the evening – crisps, nuts or chocolate. I'm trying to break the habit by eating healthier snacks and cutting down on the TV watching, too, and I'm also determined not to allow my own kids to develop the same habits, which is why I give them their after-school snacks while walking home.**"**

Lucy

"We've made it a habit to give our kids a bowl of carrot and pepper sticks just before every meal. I think they eat them without even thinking about it, now.**"**

Carol, mum to kids aged five and three

Making sure they have enough to eat

All children should have a good breakfast, every day, and this is no less important for those with an over-fondness for junk food – if they eat well and healthily first thing in the morning, they'll be less likely to have hunger pangs later and reach for the unhealthy snacks.

> Make sure that the lunches and dinners they eat are substantial enough to fill them up – just substantial in a healthy way, with roughly the right proportions of protein, carbs and vegetables.

Switch refined carbs to complex varieties wherever possible – less sugar, white bread and white rice, and more wholemeal pasta and bread; brown rice and oat-based porridge or flapjacks. All these are more satisfying as well as being more healthy. Protein is also essential for filling them up, sustaining blood sugar and boosting growth and repair, so try to ensure they have some with every meal, taking care if necessary when these are served up with rich sauces.

Keep a limit on choices

A certain amount of choice is no bad thing when it comes to encouraging healthy eating habits, as it's a positive bit of psychology – children often respond well if allowed to make some of their own decisions and have a certain amount of control over what they eat or put on their plate (or at least, if they think they've got control, which may not necessarily be the same thing!)

However, too much choice ain't great – in fact, too much choice is widely cited as one of the reasons we have a growing obesity problem in the first place. In the good old days, there just wasn't so much to choose from – kids got what they were given, and they ate it because if they didn't, they'd go hungry. Not so nowadays, when we are, probably literally, spoiled for choice.

> **Work on keeping their choices limited, at mealtimes and where snacks are concerned. Offer choice by all means if it helps you to get something good down them, but in a limited way.**

And make sure all the options are healthy ones, as there's not much point in pitching a plate of cabbage against a bowl of chips. For instance: 'do you want carrots with that, or peas? Would you like chicken or tuna in your lunch box sandwich today? Shall I put cottage cheese or baked beans on your jacket potato? A banana or a yoghurt for dessert?'

Setting the right example: why it's still the most important thing you can do!

As already discussed in chapter 3, it's up to us adults to lead the way: inevitably, a child who eats too much or has too-high a proportion of junk in their diet, has picked up those habits from their parents (though peers can also be hugely influential), or does so because they have been allowed to. So, although we've said it already, we're going to say it again: the easiest and most effective way to get your kids to eat healthily is to make it an ingrained part of your lifestyle at home, and fundamental to that is setting a good example yourselves.

> You really can't expect a child to lay off the chips and chocolate if that's what they see you eating on a regular basis.

Why it's *still* okay to indulge sometimes

Some occasions call for a bit of excess and indulgence – Christmas, Easter, and birthdays are the obvious ones but there may be many more events in the average family's year that demand a blow-out of some kind. Trouble is, if you add up these 'special' events, they come round pretty regularly, so keep an eye on how often you relax your usual standards.

And remember, you don't have to relax them completely: it doesn't make you a party pooper if you aim to be moderate when laying on a feast. For instance, there's no law that children's party food has to include six flavours of crisps, four types of biscuit, and rounded off with jelly, ice cream and cake. Focus on colours, theme and presentation instead, and you might find no-one notices you've actually put out a reasonably healthy spread. See page 105 for some tips.

When the occasion is being hosted by someone else, there's not a lot you can do about it.

> **Relax and leave them to it – a major splurge once every so often won't hurt them if they eat a balanced diet at home.**

When it comes to Easter and Christmas, there's no harm in trying to reduce the chocolate mountain a little by buying (and spread the words among relatives, too) seasonally themed non-food gifts, instead. And as for Advent calendars – well, they never used to have chocolate in them! A lovely alternative is the sort you get with little pockets, each of which can be filled with a tiny gift.

Dr Sandi says: 'There's nothing worse than the 'helicopter mum' who hovers over her child at a party, ready to whisk anything unsuitable out of their hands. At parties, I say, "Let 'em eat cake" like everyone else. As they get older the parties become less frequent, so it's a short-term concern.'

Parties that won't make them pop

- Make a healthier chocolate birthday cake that they won't even realise is healthier: try halving the amount of sugar in the recipe, and add blended stoneless prunes which don't affect the taste and actually make it more moist. Use half wholemeal and half white flour to boost the fibre content, and decorate with good quality chocolate mixed with crème fraiche, a dusting of icing sugar and chocolate buttons.

- Skewer cherry tomatoes, chunks of cucumber and cubes of cheese on cocktail sticks to make mini savoury kebabs. Make sure you keep an eye on young children if you're letting them have cocktail sticks.

- Stick to plain crisps rather than novelty varieties which have artificial flavourings and colours.

- Buy good quality sausages and cut up rather than buying the ready cooked sort which are generally higher in fat and lower in meat content.

- Serve a good selection of sandwiches with healthy fillings like cold chicken, tuna, cream cheese and egg. Shape them with a cookie cutter for added interest and try making them with one slice of wholemeal and one slice of white for added fibre.

- Have a chocolate fondue as the centrepiece and get them to use plastic forks to dip strawberries and chunks of banana and other fruits into it (careful supervision required – for obvious safety reasons).

- Add fresh fruit to jelly. (But don't serve the sweet stuff until after they've all got a few sarnies down them.)

- Substitute sorbet or frozen yoghurt for ice cream.

- Give them fruit juice diluted with sparkling mineral water, home-made milkshakes, or well-diluted high-fruit squash instead of pop.

- Splash out a bit on themed paper plates, cups and novelties like straws or blowers. They probably won't even notice what they're eating anyway!

- Don't give chocolate and sweets as prizes, or bother putting them in the party bags – kids are just as happy with rubbishy little souvenirs.

Summary

- Kids whose diets are dominated by junk food are also more likely to have health problems – even if they're not actually overweight.

- You can't control what they eat all the time, and there's no point in trying. If they have a basically healthy lifestyle at home, it won't matter much what they consume when you're not with them.

- Swap junk food for a healthier option whenever you can.

References

1   Food for the Brain child survey (2007).

Dealing with overeaters

what this chapter covers:

- Are our children eating too much?
- Does my child have a weight problem?
- Isn't it just puppy fat?
- How to put your child on a 'diet' without them realising
- Keeping control over portion sizes
- How much is too much?
- Know what they're eating
- Drinks count, too
- Are they overeating for a deeper reason?
- Avoid labels, and watch what you say
- Different issue, same rules

Are our children eating too much?

You can barely open a newspaper these days without a headline about obesity and why it's a growing problem for the population generally as well as among the younger generation. There are many and varied statistics, but whichever ones you look at, they are pretty terrifying – levels of obesity have been steadily rising in the last couple of decades and look set to continue upwards.

> **Gloomily, it's been predicted that one in three English children will be overweight or obese by 2010[1].**

When you think about it, it seems pretty obvious why this change in our bodies has impacted so significantly in recent times. Experts have been pondering and theorising about it for a while now, but what seems clear is that kids' (and, indeed adults') lifestyles are just vastly different from what they were 40 or 50 years ago. For instance:

- We use cars more and are less likely to walk when we go somewhere. Children are less likely to walk to school and, perhaps because of safety fears, less likely to play outside, climb trees, build camps and generally move around outdoors, and schools offer less PE than they used to. Preferred activities tend to be more sedentary – there's too much telly watching and computer use.

- There are many more unhealthy commercial foods available and consumption of these is ingrained in our culture.

- The ever-growing mass media and our children's exposure to them mean young people are directly targeted by those who market these products.

- Food is plentiful, available and relatively cheap so portion sizes are larger and we all eat more, generally speaking – just because we can.

Why is this 'obesity time bomb' so significant? Because of the huge risks that obesity has for our health. Growing numbers of children are developing Type 2 diabetes – previously called late onset diabetes as it did not occur until middle or old age – which is linked to being overweight. And they are at increased risk of serious health problems later in life, including heart disease, osteoarthritis, high blood pressure and certain cancers.

♨ **Dr Sandi says:** 'There's so much more choice available nowadays. There are hundreds of different varieties of chocolate bar, crisps and other snack foods. This means that we can never really tire of anything. Our bodies are designed to 'habituate' to any stimulus – put simply, this means that if we keep being exposed to the same thing, eventually it loses its appeal to us. This applies to most things and explains why a scary rollercoaster is not so scary the 10th time around. We habituate to it and get bored. The same with foodstuffs. The problem is that today, as soon as we habituate to one delicacy, we simply move on to something else – and because there are so many options out there, we never really reach saturation point. The vast array of stuff out there means that we eat more and more.'

Does my child have a weight problem?

It may seem obvious by the way they look that your child has a weight problem, but to know for sure you need to get them measured by a professional who'll either calculate their BMI (body mass index) or their body fat percentage.

There are online BMI calculators specifically designed for children (it's a more complex measurement than the fairly straightforward adult version as it has to take into account differences in age and gender), including one provided by the charity Weight Concern [www.shape-up.org/weightcon/childbmi], but your best bet is to ask a health professional such as a GP or surgery nurse to do it for you. (Weighing programmes have recently been introduced in schools, undertaken in Year 5 and Year 6, although they're not compulsory).

A visit to a sympathetic GP could also rule out a very small handful of medical reasons for a child being overweight, such as an underactive thyroid, and they should be able to provide you with some sound nutrition and dietary advice, too, or at least refer you elsewhere for more specialised help. However, if you find that you don't get the comprehensive support you need from your GP in this situation you may want to consider seeking the services of an independent nutritionist or dietitian. You can get further information about these from organisations such as the British Dietetic Association or the Nutrition Society or BANT (British Association of Nutritional Therapists). Details for both groups are listed at the back of the book.

> ☝ Dr Sandi says: 'If you do need to take a child to the doctor because you suspect they have a weight problem, the emphasis should be on health, not weight. Make it clear it's because you want them to stay healthy, not because of what they look like. Healthy eating and exercise are the issues to be flagged up, not appearance.'

Isn't it just puppy fat?

Many parents don't realise it when they have an overweight child, or else they can see they're overweight but don't really think of it as a problem. One study found that only a quarter of parents recognised the fact that their children were overweight, and that a third of mothers thought their obese child was 'just right'[2]. Some may still be caught up in that 'love 'em/feed 'em' fervour of very early childhood, when fat cheeks and chubby legs somehow validate the belief that you're doing a good job as a parent. And there may also be some 'denial' issues as a parent – if you accept that your child is fat, then you also have to accept the fact that it may be partly your fault.

Others are perhaps passing it off as 'puppy fat' which they assume they'll grow out of as they become older and taller. And, inevitably, many parents of overweight or obese children are overweight themselves and have bad eating habits and sedentary lifestyles which they pass on by example to their offspring. Recent research confirmed there is a 'fat' gene which means kids with one or more overweight parent are highly likely to have the same predisposition to put on weight[3]. But that doesn't rule environmental and lifestyle factors out of the equation – what and how we eat is still massively significant to how that genetic predisposition is expressed. All of which means that parents with a tendency to be heavy themselves need to be even more conscientious about setting a good example and encouraging healthy lifestyles than those who don't. Unfair perhaps – but then, life's like that.

As for puppy fat, well it's true that some children shed the pounds as they grow upwards. But evidence shows that if a child is still carrying so-called 'puppy fat' once they enter adolescence, the likelihood is that they will still be carrying it as an adult.[4]

However, it's important to bear in mind that a certain amount of weight gain during puberty is perfectly normal, particularly for girls, as bodies naturally change shape and fill out during this period.

" Our children have always really enjoyed their food, and to be honest, we've encouraged it – we're big eaters ourselves, and I think it always feels good to know your kids are eating well. It's only recently that it dawned on us, though, that the eldest is getting rather podgy, and the youngest is going the same way. So we've cut back on portion sizes and quietly reduced the number of cakes and biscuits we offer them. **"**

Katherine, mum to sons aged 10 and eight

" Because we're both overweight we try to give our little boy healthy choices and keep an eye on him. So although he eats a lot, it's almost always wholesome stuff. We do try to eat healthily as a family and we try to sit down together to eat at least the evening meal. But I haven't managed to diet successfully since he was born, because I don't want to pass on the wrong message to him about food. **"**

Claire, mum to a son aged three

How to put your child on a 'diet' without them realising

If you suspect your child has a weight problem or is heading that way, there are very compelling reasons why you need to do something about it. The benefit to their physical health is the most obvious – but there are also huge psychological implications for an overweight child, notably that it can affect their confidence and self-esteem.

In spite of what we've titled this section, most children shouldn't be put on 'diets', full-stop. For one thing, they are still growing and any significant reduction in their nutritional intake may affect growth or energy levels. For another, they may be more likely to develop an unhealthy relationship with food – possibly even an eating disorder – later on.

Certainly, children shouldn't ever be worried by adult preoccupations such as calorie-counting and scale-hopping, and never should they be subjected to faddy or fashionable eating plans which are based on the virtual abstention of whole food groups – in particular the sorts that banish carbs, which are particularly essential for kids because of the energy they provide.

> It's vital that an overweight child doesn't feel they are the odd one out. That way, misery lies.

So, while it's true to say that some children, if they are a long way beyond a healthy weight for their size, may need to follow a medically approved diet and exercise programme (and it goes without saying that this sort of thing should never be undertaken without supervision and guidance from a doctor or dietitian), in most cases an overweight child won't need to eat a diet that's different from anyone else's – just a moderate, sensible one which is what everyone in the family should be eating, anyway, that will help them gradually become a healthy weight for their size as they grow in height.

> **The healthiest and most effective way to help a child 'lose weight' is to make small, achievable changes to their lifestyle in a way that involves the whole family.**

KEEP CONTROL OVER PORTION SIZES

Rather than having to say 'no' to second portions for kids who need to watch their weight, offer a smaller portion in the first place, so that you can then reasonably give a second if they demand it and they're less likely to feel deprived and resentful. Steer them towards extra protein (assuming it's fairly plainly served protein such as fish or chicken, not something that's covered in a fatty cheese sauce, for example) or vegetables if they ask for more. Put these things on the table and allow them to help themselves so they can feel independent and in control. And be sensible about the amount of food you cook in the first place. If you know they adore roast potatoes and chips, just cook enough of those things to allow for a sensible portion for everyone. That way they can't have more, even if they want them.

If they're still peckish after their main course, let them have a healthy desert of fruit, yoghurt or a moderate portion of a homemade pudding such as crumble (made with a high proportion of fruit and served with Greek yoghurt or crème fraîche, this can be a perfectly healthy option for dessert). In fact, it's actually a good idea to offer something sweet after every meal to prevent sugar cravings later on.

> **It's always worth reminding a 'still hungry' child that it can take a few minutes for full feelings to hit home. Try suggesting they play a game or go in the garden for a while if they still want more food. Chances are they'll get embroiled in whatever they're doing, and realise they're replete after all.**

HOW MUCH IS TOO MUCH?

It's hard to specify exactly what a sensible portion should consist of as it varies according to age, size and energy needs.

A very general guide:

- One portion of carbs = one slice of bread OR a 30g bowl of breakfast cereal OR three small potatoes OR half a cup of cooked rice

- One portion of dairy = one yoghurt OR 2oz of cheese OR a glass of milk

- One portion of protein = two eggs OR 50g of nuts or seeds OR 75g of cooked chicken, fish or lean meat.

(Of course, none of us should be enslaved by the scales – if in doubt about portions, the 'size of the palm' analogy isn't a bad general rule to follow – and that's the size of their palm, not yours.)

Never cut back too dramatically on portion size regardless of whether or not you've got a weight problem on your hands – less than their daily needs could mean they're not getting their nutrition requirements, or enough fuel for their energy needs. Although it will vary according to age and size, average daily calorie needs for children are:

- Boy aged 4–7: 1,715 calories

- Girl aged 4–7: 1,545 calories

- Boy aged 7–10: 1,970 calories

- Girl aged 7–10: 1,740 calories

If you do need to cut back on their portion sizes, do so very gradually in small increments, adding larger amounts of fruit and vegetables to their plate to make up for it. Serve at least two sorts of vegetable with each meal and make plenty, so they've got the option of eating more if they're still hungry, and dish up starchy accompaniments like spuds in healthier ways wherever possible – for instance, mash made without butter, new rather than roast, and wedges rather than chips.

Having said all that, it's much better not to obsess about portion sizes and what sort of precise quantities of 'treat foods' they should or shouldn't eat.

> It's better to employ generous doses of common sense and take an overall view of their diet generally – as well, of course, as encouraging them to be as active as possible at the same time.

Don't put outright bans on any sort of food, however unhealthy or calorific you know they are. Even for kids with a weight problem, 'unhealthy' foods are okay in moderate quantities as part of a balanced diet. Just try not to label foods as 'unhealthy' or 'bad' because it may make them more appealing.

🍅 Sally says: 'Remember, children need good quantities of carbohydrates and fats so most adult weight-loss diets won't be suitable for them. Just shift the balance gradually over time, from saturated fats to essential fats (found in nuts, seeds and oily fish) and from refined carbohydrates to complex ones.'

KNOW WHAT THEY'RE EATING

Be aware of what you're feeding them – especially anything that's come out of a packet. There's no need to obsessively count calories for them, but do check labels and be conscious of what they're consuming. Look out for excessive amounts of fat and sugar, in particular – fortunately most manufacturers these days make this a much easier task thanks to traffic light labelling, which shows at a glance what sort of quantities are in it. Cook from scratch whenever possible – at least you know exactly what's going into it and it will invariably be healthier than your average processed commercial product, particularly if you take steps to adapt recipes by cutting the amount of fat and sugar in them or choosing alternative, healthier, ingredients.

DRINKS COUNT, TOO

Watch what they're drinking, too – lots of parents don't realise how significant drinks can be to a diet (see p.30), commercial drinks are often loaded with sugar (not to mention other nasties such as caffeine, citric acid and additives), but don't be tempted by 'diet' or 'no added sugar' versions as an alternative, as these will usually have sweeteners in them which may have health risks.

If they don't already, try and get them drinking more water – as well as being good for their overall health, it helps to keep hunger pangs at bay and dehydration can often be mistaken for hunger. Splash out, if necessary on cutely packaged mini bottles of spring water, or fun drinks containers. Serve water with ice or sliced lemon if the novelty helps.

Fruit juice diluted with sparkling water makes a refreshing alternative to fizzy drinks, or you could try offering lollies made with fruit juice. It's always worth offering a drink first when they claim to be hungry as thirst and hunger can often be confused.

EXERCISE IS KEY

We know this is a book about food, but we must also mention the vital importance of exercise, which goes hand-in-hand with a good, balanced diet for a healthy lifestyle – in fact, some experts have suggested that it's not so much the eating habits of the current generation that are to blame for the growing crisis, as the lack of activity in their lives. A child with a weight problem may need to reduce their television and computer habits, walk more (to and from school, for starters, assuming it's within walking distance) and get their booties into the great outdoors a bit more.

> **The Department of Health recommends an hour of moderate exercise, every day.**

Resist selling it as exercise, though – as with healthy eating, just make it an ordinary and enjoyable element of all your lives: walk wherever possible instead of taking the car, turn the telly off sometimes and take a tumble round the garden instead; push back the furniture and dance yourselves dizzy; go to a pub with a bouncy castle in the garden, try setting up an obstacle course or bike trail, or go for a surprise picnic after school once in a while – take friends, a selection of bats and balls, and head for the hills!

66When my daughter was younger she became bored with having to walk the dog every day so we would set up a trail of red wool tied to branches or stuck to a wall that she had to find. It was amazing how well she walked after that!99

Tracy, mum to daughters aged 13 and 11

Are they overeating for a deeper reason?

Some children may have psychological reasons for overeating, just as grown-ups do. Comfort seeking is the most obvious – they may turn to food to help them get through a difficult period in their lives such as when they're finding the going tough at school, if their parents are having relationship difficulties, or when they are being bullied (with the rather cruel consequence being a vicious circle: overweight children are often bullied or may lack confidence, and bullied or unconfident children may well turn to food for comfort).

Kids may also use food as a straightforward replacement for a loved-one who isn't always around when they wish they were.

66 I've always turned to food for comfort and as a result I've struggled to control my weight. As a child, my mum was often not back from work when I got home from school and as I wasn't allowed to cook for myself I had to wait until she got home a bit later. I think that's why I associate food with comfort. Mum died when I was 17 – ever since I've been locked in a pattern of comfort eating when alone. **99**

Daisy

Dr Sandi says: 'Eating out of the need for comfort and reassurance starts young – babies are comforted at their mother's breast and we never really lose that association between food (and mum) and comfort. As tots, it's mum who provides most of the comfort, but as they grow up, food often replaces her, in the same way that some object like a security blanket can be a substitute for mum in her absence. Food and mothers are intimately entwined for obvious reasons. So it may be that some children may turn to food because, for some reason, they can't get the comfort they need from their mother. (This does not make the mums of over-eaters bad mothers – just that an over-eating child may be seeking something that's not attainable, such as the full-time attention of their mum.) We all do this to some extent. As we grow up, we often can't access the comfort we might want from our mothers, so we may well reach for a food we love as an alternative. In fact, any parent or care-giver can have a great influence over eating habits and children's reactions to absent dads, busy dads, or bereavement can also include changing attitudes to food. Children can also overeat because of low self-esteem, or even boredom. Low self-esteem can cause them to abuse their bodies – they don't really value themselves enough to care about looking or feeling good. And boredom is a classic reason, for adults too, but probably the easiest one to solve. Finding the reason for overeating can be tricky. Your child may not know themselves, or may not want to discuss sensitive issues. It's important to look at the whole child in the context of their life to try and figure out whether they are generally happy. Find out as much as you can about their school social life, their academic ability and their general interests. This should help build a picture of a happy, fulfilled, busy child – or one who's lacking in one or more of those areas. Such a lack could be a reason for unhealthy psychological attitudes towards food.'

Avoid labels, and watch what you say

Naturally, psychology plays its part in a big way if you are trying to change the habits of an over-eater. Don't bang on about their unhealthy ways, or mention their chubby tummies. Never 'label' them in any way: you may create a subconscious urge in them to live up to their reputation.

Just as with a fussy eater – or any sort of eater, for that matter – avoid offering food as comfort to a child, and be mindful of offering it as a reward. Many experts believe it's not a good idea to elevate food to 'reward' status as it may boost its desirability and downgrade the appeal of other, more healthy foods.

Equally, don't go overboard with praise if they've eaten well and healthily or made a healthy choice over an unhealthy one – you want them to see those sorts of choices as everyday and ordinary, rather than looking to you for a huge pat on the back as though it's some great achievement when they have done so. Gentle encouragement and approval is fine, though.

🎗 Dr Sandi says: 'If they feel good from your excessive praise, the opposite side of the coin is that they feel bad when they make unhealthy choices. This can kick into a destructive self-esteem cycle – they feel that they are 'bad' and 'worthless' for eating 'bad' things.'

> **It's crucial to be sensitive if your child has an overeating or weight issue, particularly if they're the only one in the family with the problem.**

If you've decided that their eating habits need to change, introduce the changes as quietly as you can, and never cause them to feel isolated by imposing separate eating habits on them – the whole family will benefit from healthy eating, so you can feel free to make those healthy lifestyle changes across the board. You will have to be extra sensitive if you also have a fussy eater in the family. It's not unusual to have both sorts of difficult eaters sitting round one table. In fact, one is often a response to the other as the sibling of the child who gets lots of attention at the table – whether because they are fussy or because they eat too much – might react by using their own food intake to grab a slice of the attention too. You'll need to be very careful, for instance, about putting extra potatoes onto the plate of a fussy eater who'll eat little else while simultaneously trying to restrict an overeater who needs to cut down on their spuds – otherwise, you might easily leave the overeater feeling deprived and unhappy. In this situation you may need to develop a kindly dealt system of trade-offs, explaining to all concerned that the fussy eater gets extra potatoes because he's missing out on all the stuff their sibling will eat. But, generally speaking, the best way to deal with such a discrepancy is to make sure that everyone, as far as possible, eats in the same, broadly healthy, way.

> **"**My eldest started comfort eating after his dad died, and by the time I noticed, he really needed to cut down his food intake before he developed a weight problem. However, I didn't want to use the word 'diet' in front of him or give him any kind of complex about his weight. My solution was to introduce several spurious new house rules for everyone (his two brothers included), such as 'no snacking while watching television because of the spills on the sofa'.**"**
>
> *Miranda, mum to sons aged 11, nine and six*

> **Be mindful of the language you use. Never imply that they are on a 'diet'; that they need to 'watch their weight', or that a certain food is to be avoided because it's 'fattening', for example.**

At the same time, it's no bad thing for children to be exposed to positive messages about concepts such as healthy eating and moderation. Emphasise the positive rather than the negative when it comes to talking about food and diet and use simple language they can understand – so, you could perhaps talk about why nutritious foods like fruit and vegetables are good for us because the minerals and vitamins help us to ward off germs; that proteins like meat, fish and pulses will boost our muscle power, and that milk and cheese will give us nice strong bones. Let them know that treat foods like cake, chips and chocolate are okay – but are not really beneficial to us, and therefore something to be enjoyed on a less frequent basis.

Do be conscious of going overboard on the healthy eating message, though. One researcher has keyed the term 'muesli mum' when referring to mothers who take the whole healthy eating thing too far, and risk causing serious emotional and physical ill-effects to their kids. Other experts have also voiced their concern about the rise in eating disorders in ever younger children, and suggested it may be an unwanted consequence of healthy eating campaigns. Although these disorders are still extremely rare among children, it's a link that may be worth bearing in mind.

🐱 **Dr Sandi says:** 'It's vital to watch what you say to a child with a weight problem. The most innocuous comment can trigger an eating disorder (although these are rarely caused by a desire to lose weight in itself and are usually tied up with self-esteem or control issues). Equally you need to be mindful of how you treat such a child in comparison to siblings who don't have the same problem – it would be awful to allow one child pudding, but the other only fruit. Admittedly this can be tricky if the sibling is underweight and could do with the extra calories: the answer may be that for five teatimes out of seven you give them both fruit, and then, on the other two evenings, you let them both have the pudding. It's essential that the overweight child feels as secure and happy about themselves as possible. Never make them feel that your love is conditional – in other words, contingent on them losing weight. This might be the furthest thing from your mind but your child might feel that they will not be loved if they are fat, or that you prefer their thinner sibling.'

Different issue, same rules

You may think that a child who's an overeater will require a completely different set of guidelines from the difficult eaters we looked at in the chapter 4. But in fact, many of the rules are the same – your ultimate aim, after all, is to have a child who eats well, and healthily.

The following points have all been made before in this book – and all apply here, too:

- Eat together as a family, at the table, as often as possible.

- Don't use food for comfort. Be careful about using it as a reward.

- Set the right example.

- Stick to regular mealtimes, and never skip meals.

- Get them interested in (good) food.

- Chill out: there's absolutely nothing to be gained by getting uptight about it.

This goes too for the child with a weight problem. They are perfectly entitled to indulge at parties once in a while, assuming they're eating a balanced diet at home. And you can always minimise the damage by lining their stomachs well beforehand. If it's an afternoon party, for example, give them a good, healthy lunch, and then you know that when they're cramming the E-numbers in and bouncing off the walls with a sugar rush later that day, you'll have done the best you can. Swipe that party bag from them as soon as you can – the sweeties and cake can be put in the cupboard for another day (or, if you have a fighting chance of getting away with it, thrown away altogether).

Summary

- Obesity and overeating are growing problems for modern children, who tend to lead more sedentary lives than they used to and eat more unhealthy foods.

- Children who are obese or overweight are more at risk of a range of medical conditions and may suffer emotionally, too.

- Parents of children with a weight problem don't always realise it.

- In most cases, an overweight child will not need to 'diet', just undergo a change of lifestyle.

- Overweight children shouldn't be subjected to a change of lifestyle alone – the whole family should be included.

- Keep an eye on portion size and the amount of 'seconds' given to children who are overweight or who have a tendency to overeat.

- Be label aware, as there can be a huge amount of extra sugar, fat and other undesirable ingredients in prepackaged food.

- Remember that many drinks are also high in sugar, so keep an eye on these.

- The right attitude is vital when you have a child who needs to watch their weight. It's crucial that they don't feel hurt or isolated by the problem.

- Children who overeat may do so because of an underlying emotional issue.

References

1 Department of Health, 2006.

2 Alison Jeffery et al: Overweight families – unaware and unconcerned. British Medical Journal (2005).

3 Wardle J, et al: Evidence for a strong genetic influence on childhood adiposity despite the force of obesogenic environment, American Journal of Clinical Nutrition (2008).

4 Wardle J et al: Development of adiposity in adolescence: five-year longitudinal study of an ethnically and socio-economically diverse sample of young people in Britain, BMJ (2006).

8

Children with special dietary needs

what this chapter covers:

- When a special diet might be required
- Food allergies and intolerances
- Autistic spectrum
- Hyperactivity
- Why label awareness is vital
- Foods that are believed to affect children's behaviour...and how to avoid them
- How the rest of the family can help
- Helping them to help themselves
- Putting it into perspective

When a special diet might be required

Having a child with a special dietary need can bring a new and even trickier dimension to dealing with a difficult eater, and removing or avoiding one or more particular foods will usually require a parent to be sensitive, firm, diligent and ultra-organised – on a permanent basis. It's by no means impossible, but it can be hard work, as you learn – sometimes on a trial and error basis which foods are okay and which aren't – and in the process, convince your child that sticking with their special diet is entirely in their own interests. There are a number of reasons why children may need to follow a special diet which we will cover in this chapter.

FOOD ALLERGIES AND INTOLERANCES

An allergy is the immune system's response to a usually harmless food or substance which it perceives as being dangerous, resulting in one or more of a wide range of physical symptoms. The mildest and commonest of these may be runny noses, rashes, coughing, sneezing and sore eyes. Most severe – and thankfully very unusual – is anaphylaxis, which involves a rapid drop in blood pressure and narrowing of the airways and, without prompt medical response, can be fatal.

> Genuine food allergies are in fact pretty unusual, although they are more common in young children (who in the vast majority of cases, will grow out of them before they reach school age).

Research findings vary – studies carried out in 2001 by the British Nutrition Foundation concluded that true food allergy affects just 1%–2% of children (and less than 1% of adults), while a 2007 report by a team at the University of Portsmouth found that 5%–6% of children are affected. Research also shows that a much higher percentage of parents believe their kids to have an allergy – so clearly, it's perceived to be a worse problem than it actually is.

> The most common 'trigger' foods in children are citrus fruits, cows' milk, eggs, nuts, shellfish, soya, tomatoes and wheat. But allergies can be hard to diagnose, not least because they are often confused with food intolerance (see below).

There's little in the way of treatment for allergies, so the main way to help a child who's suffering is to establish what the trigger foods are, usually with the aid of a blood or skin-prick test carried out by an allergist or paediatrician.

Asthma, eczema and hayfever are allergy-related conditions and their symptoms can also be triggered or exacerbated by eating certain foods. Some sufferers of eczema, for example, find life is easier when they avoid dairy products as they can cause an inflammatory response – it's always worth trying cutting out these foods to see if it makes a difference (and it may not), but only ever under medical or nutritional guidance and with careful attention to the correct alternatives.

Intolerance to a food means the body has difficulty in digesting something causing a range of symptoms which, although unpleasant – bloating and diarrhoea for example – are unlikely to be harmful. Common foods that cause intolerance include lactose (the naturally occurring sugar found in cows' milk), wheat and gluten. Some people find that chemical preservatives and additives produce undesirable symptoms, more usually due to a toxic reaction, rather than an immune response.

An overgrowth of yeast in the gut is believed by some experts to be an underlying cause of some food allergies and intolerances – if 'friendly' bacteria are low due to stress, infections or medications such as steroids or antibiotics, then the gut becomes inflamed and can break down, making it 'leaky'. This can allow food proteins to cross over into the bloodstream in larger than normal particles and set off an immune response resulting in intolerances to certain foods, the most common of which are wheat or cows' milk products.

> Probiotics can help to control the situation but won't eradicate infections, stop intolerances or heal the gut in the long term.

Intolerances are more common than allergies, but still less common than many people think – between 8% and 12% of children (depending on which research you read) are thought to be affected.

AUTISTIC SPECTRUM

Autism is a hugely complex biological disorder which causes a wide range of physical and behavioural problems. Some parents of children with autistic spectrum disorders believe that careful monitoring of their diet can significantly improve an autistic child's behaviour, due to a possible link between autism and digestive problems.

> It's thought that removing gluten (the protein found in wheat, rye, barley and oats) and/or casein (a protein found in milk) can help.

Children with autism can also sometimes display unusual eating habits and rituals which may be mistaken for ordinary fussy eating. For instance, they may only eat beige or green food; want either dry food like crackers, or wet food such as milk or yoghurt; or they may refuse to have anything on their plate touch anything else, or refuse to touch it with their fingers. (However, a child displaying one or more of these tendencies is by no means necessarily autistic.)

HYPERACTIVITY

While there is little definitive evidence to show that the group of conditions encompassing Attention Deficit Hyperactivity Disorder (ADHD), Attention Deficit Disorder (ADD) and hyperactivity has links to diet, many parents with a hyperactive child and some practitioners believe there are.

> **The main suspects seem to be sugar, salicylates (naturally occuring compounds that occur in certain fruit and vegetables), a lack of fatty acids in the diet, blood sugar imbalances and toxic metals.**

Some artificial additives in a child's diet are believed by many to be influential on behaviour and worsen hyperactivity. (See p.182)

Why label awareness is vital

Parents of children with special dietary needs must become label detectives. You will need to double-check the ingredients of everything. Many common problem foods such as wheat, dairy and soya can find their way into the most unexpected of products, and you also need to know any other less obvious names the banned food masquerades under. Sugar, for example, has several dozen different aliases.

An extremely useful booklet for helping to make sense of what goes into food and what it's called is the FINDOUT additive decoder, published by Foresight, the pre-conceptual care association. You can order one from the Foresight website, at www.foresight-preconception.org.uk.

There'll always be some kind of safe alternative to any problem food, so you'll need to know what these are and how to get hold of them. In some cases, the most palatable option may be to make it yourself (wheat-free bread, for example), so you may well have to be prepared to roll your sleeves up in the kitchen a bit more. And supermarkets are increasingly stocking a wide range of gluten and wheat-free products to cater for people with allergies and intolerances.

Good organisation is also key – you may need them to take a packed lunch or snack with them wherever they go so they will always have an alternative to hand should it be necessary.

Always seek advice from a GP or nutritionist before removing any foods permanently from your child's diet. They could be missing out on important nutrients and you'll need to know what to give them as an alternative.

> **"**One thing that's helped my son cope with the diet restrictions is to always have decent alternatives tucked away in every coat/ bag /glove compartment so that substitutions can take place immediately. We also save up all the rubbish he's given (in party bags, and from older relatives who refuse to believe me when I say that the synthetics in foods affect his behaviour) and make an enormous gunk with it adding baked beans, mud, dead worms, and have a good play with it. One got left in the cellar for a month – it became nice and furry.**"**

Chez, mum to sons aged six and two

Foods that are believed to affect children's behaviour... and how to avoid them

Sugar

Where's it found?

In a massive range (and often in huge quantities) of products such as cakes, biscuits, confectionery, pudding, cereals, and drinks such as squash or pop. Some of these things contain shocking amounts of the white stuff, as a quick label check will reveal. The average can of cola, for example, has 35g.

What does it do?

Many parents, having carried out their own, highly unscientific but nevertheless convincing studies on their own kids, will tell you that an overload of sugar makes their kids noisy, naughty, or moody. That's because sugar is a short-lived stimulant, much like caffeine. It elevates blood sugar which results in increased activity levels, with a resulting slump when the glucose has been dispersed. But while a slice of cake (or a cup of coffee) generally amounts to a useful energy boost for your average adult, children are more susceptible to the stimulant effect and, for some, it can induce hyperactivity. Most kids can tolerate small amounts of sugar but the modern diet contains so much, often hidden, that it builds up, and the effect is often cumulative. And sugar has other health risks, too, as it's linked to immune suppression, tooth rot, obesity and diabetes.

How to avoid it

- Keep sugary products to a minimum and avoid in large doses.

- Give diluted fruit juices and water instead of fizzy drinks.

- When checking labels watch out for all the other names that sugar can go by, such as sucrose, dextrose, glucose, and inverted sugar syrup.

- Bake your own cakes and treats where possible and try halving sugar in all recipes.

- Try to keep sweet things for after a meal which will

lessen any effect, or serve with some protein, fibre or fat alongside it to help slow down the release of the glucose. (For example, serve fruit with natural yoghurt, honey on wholemeal bread, or include a glass of milk with a biscuit.)

Artificial additives

Colourings, preservatives, and flavour enhancers, also known sometimes as E-numbers.

Where are they found?

In countless numbers of food products. Food additives are given an 'E-number' by EU food regulators, which means they are deemed safe. Most of them are indeed harmless, but there's mounting feeling that some of them are not.

What do they do?

If anti-additive campaigners are correct, they are linked to the behaviour of hyperactive children (and may also cause or exacerbate physical conditions such as rashes, gastric upset and asthma in some children). It's controversial because there's not much in the way of conclusive research findings on the subject. However, there's masses of anecdotal evidence that there is a link, and researchers at the university of Southampton recently came to the significant conclusion that certain mixes of a handful of artificial colourings, when combined with the artificial preservative Sodium Benzoate, could be linked to a negative effect on children's behaviour. As a result the Food Standards Agency now advises parents of kids who show signs of hyperactivity that they might want to eliminate the specific offenders from their children's diet. They are:

- Yellow food colourings

- Tartrazine (E102)

- Sunset yellow (E110)

- Quinoline yellow (E104)

- Red food colourings

- Carmoisine (E122)

- Allura red (E129)

- Ponceau 4R (E124)

Between them they are found in more than a thousand products (including a number of over-the-counter medicines). A new European ruling means manufacturers will have to include a warning about possible adverse effects on the label – until then it's a case of reading the small print. You can also check out the Food Commission's Action on Additives campaign website (www.actiononadditives.com), which has a comprehensive list of products containing the additives pinpointed by the Southampton researchers. Campaigners say there are also many other artificial additives in our foods which may cause problems, such as brilliant blue (E133) and Monosodium Glutamate (MSG, or E621), which is not recommended for children under three, in any case. The Hyperactive Children's Support Group publishes a list of all those additives they recommend be avoided (you'll find details for this and Action on Additives in the back of the book).

How to avoid them

- Give your kids fresh foods and meals and snacks prepared from scratch, wherever possible.

- When you do buy commercial products, check the labels. Of course, this isn't always possible because you can't always be hovering over your kids and not all the food we eat (ice cream from a vendor, for example) comes with a label on it.

Artificial sweeteners

Such as aspartame, saccharin, sorbitol, acesulfame-K.

Where are they found?

These are also a form of additives and are used by manufacturers to replace sugar in many drinks and other sweet products as they are lower in calories and kinder to teeth than sugar. However (as well as causing some other health concerns) some parents suspect they may affect behaviour, so they're not a particularly useful alternative for children affected by sugar.

What do they do?

As with artificial additives, they are believed by some people to be linked to hyperactive behaviour in kids.

How to avoid them

- Check the labels. In particular, watch out for the words 'no added sugar' – this usually means they have sweeteners, instead.

> **NB: Always, always seek the advice of a doctor or a qualified nutritionist or dietitian before making any major changes to your child's diet.**

How the rest of the family can help

Just because you have one child with a special dietary need, doesn't mean you don't have one or more others who are perfectly able to eat anything and everything without any adverse consequences for their health or behaviour.

It's helpful and supportive if all other members of the family can be party to food bans at the same time, wherever possible. Equally, it's not really fair to expect children with perfectly normal dietary needs to miss out on anything – and a realistic necessity for a child with a problem to learn and accept that there's something a little bit different about them, and that they need to accept it because life, unfortunately, is like that.

> ☺ **Dr Sandi says:** 'I think it's good, ideally, to have the whole family adopt the 'restricted' diet, but this is not always practical (or, indeed, healthy). I think it depends a lot on what the foodstuff is – I don't see why a whole family can't avoid cola since it has no benefits anyway. But a child who is lactose intolerant shouldn't prevent others drinking milk, because of the obvious health benefits of milk. A severe and potentially dangerous allergy to something like peanuts may well require the whole family to avoid them too, anyway, and that's fair enough – you'll just have to explain to everyone why and what the consequences would be. Obviously wherever possible you should seek out and give alternatives to the affected child.'

66 My Asperger's son's behaviour is badly affected by too much wheat and too much sugar in his diet – his behaviour immediately after drinking cola has to be seen to be believed. We banned it before he was three (by which time he'd only ever drunk it about twice, but the effect was

obvious). Last summer he persuaded me to let him try it again (he was 10). After the first glass he was fine so I stupidly let him have a second. Half an hour later one of his brothers said something that upset him (for no good reason) and he shrieked solidly for the next 20 minutes. At the end of 20 minutes he stopped dead, went quiet for about 10 minutes, and then apologised very sweetly to everyone – and agreed that he wasn't ready for cola yet. Wheat causes more sustained stress in him and even more outbursts. So we only allow it in moderate quantities and don't keep bread in the house – we've found rice cakes to be a pretty good alternative.

None of the children are allowed cola or sweet fizzy drinks, which has never been a problem. Oddly, my Asperger's son has always politely turned down cola when offered it away from home (I've been told this by other parents), which is uncharacteristically well-behaved of him.**"**

Miranda, mum to sons aged 11, nine and six

🍅 **Sally says:** 'When you have a child who cannot eat a certain something for the sake of their own health, you have to explain honestly and sensitively why, within their age limit of comprehension. It can help to use positive language, letting them know they are 'special' rather than different, and helping them to understand that there is a good reason for it – for instance, that it will help stop their headaches or tummy pains. I'm constantly amazed at how well parents cope in this situation. Most of them dread it to start with, but succeed in the end.'

"Life can be difficult for my son, who has coeliac disease – a serious medical condition caused by a sensitivity to gluten – and has been on a strict gluten-free diet since he was one. But at least he's never really known any different. He's very good about his condition (helped by the fact his dad has it too). Eating out, birthday parties, treats at school, and shopping can all be very hard. At parties, he has to take his own packed meal with him – I normally try and ask the parent what they will have so that I can try and find gluten-free alternatives to go in his lunch box. He can get quite upset about this especially when it comes to birthday cake, but we just have to remind him that his tummy is very special and he has to take extra care of it. We also make sure he has some gluten-free biscuits in a safe place at school, so that he can have a treat when the other children do. I also have a younger son who is not a coeliac and therefore can eat whatever he wants, which can cause some difficulties as he doesn't really understand why he can't share his food with his older brother. However, the majority of what we eat as a family is gluten-free. It's easier that way."

Caroline, mum to sons aged six and three

Helping them to help themselves

It's all very well keeping a close eye on a child with a special dietary need when they're very young and you're always with them. But there'll come a time when they have to take off on their own two feet and cope with their dietary issues alone, so passing on the knowledge and information they need to deal with them is vital from the start.

Even very young children from toddling onwards can be gently encouraged to recognise a problem food (at least in its most obvious forms) and to avoid it. Work on ways of passing on the information they need in a non-alarmist way – you need them to be alert but you don't want to fill them with fear: keep up a gentle dialogue with them so it goes in and you may want to check labels together, once they're old enough to make any sense of them.

> **Many parents are surprised by how accepting children can be of a food ban and how they are able to cope perfectly well in a social or other situation when their parents aren't around.**

As you can't very well follow them around 100% of the time, it's a case of learning how to let go. It goes without saying that school staff or any other sort of care-givers must be given comprehensive instruction, too.

✿ **Dr Sandi says:** 'It's difficult, but many parents find that their children are surprisingly accepting of their condition and will happily stick to their dietary requirements when out, even when they're at parties and their parents aren't around. Most seem to happily tell their hosts what they can and can't have.'

"Too many E-colourings can turn my boys into Tasmanian Devils. They are generally really good about avoiding them as they've now realised the consequences will get them told off, and I'm starting to teach the older one to read the names of the natural colourings that they are allowed, so he can check labels for himself. Most parties are actually okay, as they either take the coloured bits off (Smarties, icing and so on) or just stick to plain chocolate biscuits. It can be difficult for them when children take birthday sweets into school – mostly they accept they aren't allowed certain sweets but occasionally it causes a strop. I keep chocolate handy, as an alternative just in case, and so the situation is usually easily resolved.

Both of them question what I say all the time: 'Why can't I have it? Can I have this? Can't I just have a little bit?' and, most commonly, 'Why don't they make things without colourings in them?' I just explain that because not everyone reacts to colourings, others can have things they can't. And that the people who make sweets are silly!

I strongly believe that honesty is the best policy and that it's better to explain why they can't have it rather than just banning it from the house."

Louise, mum to sons aged six, five and two

"My youngest has problems with additives and when she goes to parties she always takes her own drink in a special flask, and knows exactly what she can and can't eat. I always feed her well before she goes, and she never seems that bothered by it. The fun of a party is in the games and the other children. I think it's we mothers who tend to obsess about what they might be missing out on."

Tania, mum to daughters aged 13 and nine

"Unfortunately my little girl, who has multiple allergies, already understands when I say, 'You can't have that because it will hurt your tummy'. She knows from experience how much pain the trigger foods cause and so she isn't really tempted. The only time I have problems is when all the children are having the same foods except for her. She then clearly feels left out and hurt, like it's a game and she's not included, so there are certain situations I try to avoid, such as Easter Egg hunts. She's the same as any other child and she wants to be included and liked."

Pippa, mum to a daughter aged two

Putting it into perspective

When all's said and done, a dietary special need is not the end of the world and will usually be manageable, given the right attitude and information. There is sometimes a tendency in parents to create more of a special need than is actually there, and also, sometimes, an opportunity (created by their parents) for a child to do so. But even where there's a very genuine problem, it will only be exacerbated by the anxious hovering of a worried parent.

> **A relaxed outlook is almost always best.**

Summary

- Children with a special need require especially sensitive handling.

- Allergies, autism and hyperactivity are among the special needs that most commonly require special diets.

- If you have a child with a special dietary need, you'll need to be constantly vigilant about what they eat.

- You'll also need to be able to read and understand food labels, and have a good understanding of what the alternatives are.

- The best way to deal with a child with a special dietary need is to be honest and upfront about the foods they cannot have.

- It's a good idea to arm them with the knowledge they need as early as is feasible – but in such a way that does not cause them anxiety or alarm.

- Where possible, it helps if the whole family can follow the same diet. If this is too difficult, the child with the special need must be helped to understand they are different. They usually can!

- Keeping perspective on the situation is vital.

9

Frequently asked questions and answers

what this chapter covers:

- Babies and weaning
- Difficult eaters
- Junk food junkies and overeaters
- Attitudes to diet and body image
- Food and nutrition, in general

We've found that the same questions seem to keep cropping up from parents concerned about food issues with their children. Here, we address the most common ones.

Babies and weaning

Q: When is it okay to let babies feed themselves? I always worry about mine choking.

Sally says: As soon as your baby wants to! You can begin to give first finger foods from around seven months and they will generally start to show an interest in independent feeding from then on, once they're sitting up in a highchair and their ability to grip small objects between their fingers begins to develop. It can take a while for them to get used to this new way of eating and they probably won't get much down the hatch for a while, but they'll have fun – try offering morsels such as pieces of banana, rice cakes, cooked carrot, cucumber and grated cheese. Now is also the time to start experimenting with a good range of different coloured cooked and raw fruit and vegetables (avoiding those that may cause allergies or be difficult to digest, such as berries and citrus fruits).

At some point they'll reach out to grab their spoon from you in a bid to give cutlery a whirl – dress them in the biggest bib you can find, put a cloth on the floor, and stand well back!

Never leave a young child unattended when eating, though, because of the risk of choking. If your baby does start to gag or seems to be choking, try not to panic and give them a few moments to cough up the offending item – they will virtually always manage to do this on their own.

If they are still struggling and seem unable to cough, cry or breath, dial 999 first, then lay them face down along your left forearm with their head low, supporting their jaw with your hand. Give five firm slaps on their back, between their shoulder blades. If this doesn't help, you can try chest thrusts: give five sharp downward thrusts on their middle chest bone and repeat this cycle up to three times, checking their mouth after each attempt. Don't be tempted to turn your baby upside down and shake to remove a blockage as this could be harmful. (NB it's best to be trained in first aid before attempting these techniques. If any any doubt, simply dial 999 and wait for help to arrive.)

Q: Do I really need to cook my baby's food from scratch? Sometimes it seems that life's too short to purée veg and fill up ice cube trays. I always give her the good quality, organic brands of commercial baby food. Is that so bad?

🍒 Sally says: There's not much doubt that home cooking is best, so aim to give them as much as you can manage. Endlessly cooking, puréeing, and filling sterilised containers can seem like a thankless task, it's true, but one way of making life easier on yourself here is by setting aside unsalted portions of appropriate food from the family's meals whenever possible.

Once they're a month or so into weaning, you don't even need to get a blender out – you can just mash with a fork. Fresh, high-quality shop-bought baby foods can of course be a good alternative when you just don't have the time, and in fact there are some very good ones available now in the chiller cabinets, such as Organix, Ella's Kitchen, or Little Dish, so if you're checking the labels and you're satisfied with what's in them, carry on.

Q: We eat lots of curries. Can I give some to my toddler?

Sally says: There's no reason why babies and toddlers can't have curries – children bought up in many ethnic households are usually given them from the start, after all. Indeed, they will often relish the strong flavours, and it's great to start them off with a broad outlook on food (even if they do go on to refuse some things when they're a bit older).

Start with something very mild such as a korma, adding small quantities of curry spices such as cumin, ground coriander, garam masala and turmeric.

Do bear in mind that very strong flavours like chilli can cause colicky pains and diarrhoea so may be best avoided altogether for children under two. If you've never served them up before, introduce spicy foods slowly, and not too often to begin with.

Difficult eaters

Q: Mealtimes are so stressful at our house. My daughter, who's four, refuses to eat a majority of the things I make for her and won't respond to any amount of encouragement or cajoling. Sometimes she pretends to be eating by filling her mouth with food which she stores in her cheeks for up to 10 minutes before spitting it out some-where after she's left the table. It's driving me mad. What can I do?

Dr Sandi says: This kind of secretive behaviour may be a consequence of too much pressure from you, so maybe you need to lower the ante a bit. Don't try and cajole her into eating, just stay calm and quietly let her know she can leave food if she really doesn't want it. Don't let her have anything other than a very simple, healthy snack such as fruit until the next meal, and then stay calm during that one, too. If mealtimes become less of a big deal for you, they'll become less of a big deal for her, too.

Q: My son has a very limited intake of fruit and vegetables. He'll eat apples and bananas, and peas and carrots. He also drinks orange juice. But I worry this isn't a broad enough range. Should I?

Ⓢ Sally says: Your son sounds as if he has a reasonable range and intake. It could be better, but he's unlikely to come to harm.

If you're really concerned, you could try adding variation by including some different sorts of fruit and veg to well-blended smoothies, soups or pasta sauces – just be sure not to lie about what you've included if challenged, which might make him suspicious of everything else you give him.

He'll probably get a bit more adventurous as he gets older. In the meantime, reassure yourself with the knowledge that it could be a lot worse. Some kids won't eat any veg at all!

Q: I don't like my son going to friends' houses for tea because he's so fussy. Am I worrying unnecessarily?

Ⓢ Dr Sandi says: Yes, let him go to tea at other people's houses – chances are, he won't behave as he does at home and you might even be surprised by what he eats while there, especially if the friend he's with is a good eater and sets a good example. Avoid saying anything to him about it before he goes, but you could quietly ask the parent what he ate afterwards. Even if it turns out to be absolutely nothing, it's not going to matter much for one day.

Q: I'm seriously concerned about the amount of food my five-year-old daughter is eating. There are days when she eats nothing more than bread and a yoghurt, although other days are better. I'm convinced it must be affecting her health. My GP says I shouldn't worry and that she'll grow out of it, but it's keeping me awake at night. Is my GP right – or should we see a specialist?

☺ Sally says: It sounds as though she's an ordinary fussy eater, rather than a child with a serious eating problem. If your GP has checked her over and is satisfied that her growth, development or general health is not affected, and if she seems to have plenty of energy and enthusiasm for life, then your GP is probably right that you don't need to worry. Most young children eat erratically, stocking up food in reserve rather like snakes, so they will eat more some days than others. It's very normal. Try and look at what she's consuming over the course of a week or two rather than a day at a time, and you may find it reassuring.

She may well begin to change her eating habits soon as she starts to mix more with other children and grows more open-minded about food. If things haven't changed much in another six months, though, you may want to return to your GP for another check-up, or perhaps seek an assessment with a nutritional therapist.

Q: Why does my six-year-old refuse to eat things she liked perfectly well before? It makes me think she's just being difficult and I tell her she must eat it because I know she likes it. Am I right?

🍎 Dr Sandi says: Well, maybe she is being difficult or maybe she genuinely has gone off it. It doesn't really matter – the point is that mealtimes should never become a battleground. Adults go off things too, especially if we have them a lot – and let's face it, when our child likes something, we tend to overdose them on it. It's normal to become bored with something we once loved – it's all part of nature's way of getting us to eat a varied diet. Whether she does or doesn't like it any more, you will have to grin and bear it and give her something else. Chances are, she'll rediscover it later on.

Another technique is to try 'reverse psychology'. Tell her she can't have that any more because she doesn't like it. This is far more likely to get her to change her mind than trying to encourage her to eat it.

Q: It drives me crazy when my four-year-old daughter won't eat her meals and I regularly lose my temper over it. If she does it to wind me up, she's extremely successful. Any tips on helping me to deal with this?

🍎 Dr Sandi says: You need to chill here. Okay, I know this is (a lot) easier said than done but it really is the only answer. Of course, the issue of why she won't eat her meals (and what exactly that means – will she not eat any of them – or just bits?) is important and worth giving some attention to first. Perhaps she is just trying to wind you up, but why? Does she get enough attention from you? Is she looking for some way of exerting control in her life? Is anything else going on in the background – new sibling, parental split etc? Or could she be testing the limits of your love for her? Perhaps she wants to see how angry you will get before you reject her.

The best strategy is to give her lots of love and attention (generally, not just at mealtimes), try to give her foods she enjoys (within reason), give her limited choices (such as carrots or peas?), involve her in food preparation and shopping where possible, and cut down on snacking. Then you will have to pretend to be relaxed about whether she eats what is offered or not. A lot of parenting involves acting and your acting skills may be called upon here. If she realises that she won't get the big reaction from you, she might just not bother seeking it. And, if she is not attention-seeking, but simply a poor eater, your being relaxed (or at least appearing to be) is far healthier for her in the long-term than flying off the handle which is invariably counter-productive.

If you really can't control your temper sometimes, then leave the dining room and take a few moments to get a grip and try to put some perspective on things. Remind yourself that even if she doesn't eat anything at all at this meal, it's not going to affect her health. As the saying goes, she'll eat when she's hungry.

Dealing with food junkies and overeaters

Q: I'm trying to cut down on the amount of junk my children eat. It's proving hard, though, as I've let them get into the habit of eating whatever they want. How can I change their eating habits without them hating me?

🖐 **Dr Sandi says:** Actually, you can show them just how much you love them by making these changes – done in the right way, they will love you right back, not hate you for it. The right way is to be moderate, not fundamentalist about it, to provide delicious alternatives, and to reinforce the message about why you are making these changes (that is, that you care about them). Make the changes gradually and involve them where possible in food buying and preparation.

Q: I caught my 10-year-old daughter binging on chocolate stolen from my cupboard. Should I be worried?

🖐 **Dr Sandi says:** Not if it's a one-off. However, it might make you want to reassess your attitude towards 'forbidden' treats. Did she nick it because chocolate is such a rare event in your house? If you are being too strict with the treat control, perhaps she is reacting against this. Of course, it is not just the bingeing that is the issue here, but the stealing. At 10, she might just have acted on impulse – she stumbled across your hidden stash and couldn't resist. But the 'crime' of stealing what is not hers must be dealt with here, too.

Q: My eldest son has a slight weight problem and our doctor has advised us to watch what he eats. His two younger sisters are fine, though, and I don't see why they should miss out. How can I deal with this situation fairly?

Dr Sandi says: You should treat all your kids the same and make sure they all eat healthily. Try not to think of it in terms of the younger ones 'missing out' by having to change their diet – instead, think of it as them missing out by not changing.

Weight is not the only indicator of a poor diet – kids can be slim but develop unhealthy eating attitudes that can rear their ugly heads later on. It would be cruel to your girls not to allow them the chance to improve their diet too. Don't cut out treats altogether for anyone, just make sure they're carefully limited. And be sure to watch what you say in front of him – don't talk about him being overweight, or having a problem which his sisters don't. Just talk in positive terms about the whole family taking a healthier approach to life.

Attitudes to diet and body image

Q: My nine-year-old daughter told me she hates her fat stomach and wants to go on a diet. She's a perfectly normal size and shape, with the tiniest of pot bellies. What should I say to her?

✍ *Dr Sandi says:* She needs to be 'inoculated' against the disease of weight obsession. Talk to her about healthy bodies and why it's beneficial to be in good proportion height/weight-wise. Then, explain why society is so obsessed with weight and how harmful this is to young girls. The best approach is to take an 'emperor's new clothes' view – the idea is that only silly girls will obsess about their weight and want to diet, savvy ones will see straight away that this emperor is naked and worthless.

Hopefully, she will want to be a savvy girl who sees through the superficiality of weight obsession.

Q: I've been advised by my doctor to lose a few stone, so I'm on a diet. I don't want this to affect my kids' attitude towards food. What should I do?

✍ *Dr Sandi says:* Don't mention the D-word (diet). Don't moan about what you can't eat and don't obsess over it. Emphasise the positives ('ooh, delicious apples!') and don't express guilt over 'forbidden treats'. Carry on eating with the family whenever possible, and don't make a big deal about what you are or are not eating. Hopefully you're on a sensible, healthy eating based weight loss plan and not doing anything silly. Exercise is the best way to burn off unwanted calories, anyway, so get out and about as much as possible – and take the kids with you.

Q: My partner is very overweight and, although they are perfectly fine now, I'm worried my kids may eventually go the same way. What can I do to prevent that?

🍅 Dr Sandi says: Your partner should lose weight for his own sake, of course, but either way, a healthy lifestyle is needed across the whole family. This includes diet and exercise, without referring to any weight-loss needs at all. There are, of course, reasons to worry about your kids following your partner – they may be genetically disposed to weight gain, or they may copy his lifestyle. Either way, the best way to counter any such influence is a holistic approach involving a good hard look at your entire lifestyle.

Q: My kids make fun of a 'fat kid' at school. How can I change their attitude without condoning the size of him, which clearly isn't healthy?

🍅 Dr Sandi says: First and foremost, this is about teaching tolerance and acceptance of other people. Just as adults have a tendency to lay the blame over fat adults ('they're lazy, they eat too much'), so kids assume that the 'fat kid' must be lazy and/or greedy. You need to explain that this may not be the case at all and point out that many overweight people have a reason for their weight problems.

Either way, the emphasis should be on the feelings of this individual who is still a person who can be hurt by unkind comments. Help them see the world from the other kid's viewpoint – perhaps one of your own kids has something different about them that could be picked on by their mates – maybe they wear glasses, have red hair, are tall, small etc.

Try to get them to imagine how they would feel to be bullied over this. And if they try to argue that 'me wearing glasses is not my fault – Harry being fat is his fault' aim to minimise any blame and emphasise the possible role of genetics, hormones etc (even if you secretly agree that the kid eats too much).

Food and nutrition, in general

Q: I've heard that essential fatty acids are really important for good health. How can I get some of them into my kids?

⏰ Sally says: This can be tricky, as the very foods that con-tain essential fatty acids (EFAs) are likely to be the ones they won't touch or are allergic to, including oily fish, nuts, seeds and leafy green veg.

Fish cakes or fish pie made with canned or fresh salmon or mackerel, or fresh tuna, are almost always popular, and a good way to make green leafy veg palatable is to add it very thinly sliced to stir fries. Try offering small bowls of unsalted nuts or seeds as a snack, too – you can really boost their taste by toasting them in a dry frying pan. They also make a nice crunchy addition to bread or rolls, if you've ever considered baking your own.

If you're really struggling and you're worried about their lack of EFAs, disguise may be your best option. You could try grinding nuts or seeds (use a pestle and mortar, or invest in a little electric coffee grinder – also very useful for grinding dry herbs and spices) and sprinkling them over or into any food where they're likely to be undetected, or you could try adding small amounts of linseed, flaxseed, walnut or rapeseed oils to your cooking.

If all else fails, you can give them a short-term boost with fish oil supplements, which are widely available from large chemists and health food shops.

Q: I want to give my family home-cooked meals, but I just don't have much time to get dinner on the table by the time I'm in from work. What's the answer?

🍅 **Sally says:** Planning ahead really helps. Write a menu plan before going to do the weekly shop and put it on the fridge so you can stick to it, then buy what you need accordingly – there's less waste that way, too. Shopping online is a good time-saver and ensures you've always got something in.

Make good use of your freezer and store cupboards: have a selection of potential meals in both, permanently. If you're cooking over the weekend, make more than you need and keep the rest for another time – one-pot basics such as tomato or bolognese sauces, chillis or casseroles freeze well. Get them out the night before to defrost thoroughly (so, a bit more planning ahead required), heat up thoroughly on the hob, and serve with rice or pasta, which only take 10 minutes to cook.

Slow cookers are a great piece of kitchen equipment for working parents – you can sling the ingredients in first thing in the morning, turn it on, and eat it as soon as you're all in.

Finally, never forget that you only need 20 minutes and fairly minimum effort to rustle up a nutritious tea from scratch: if time and inclination are truly in short supply sometimes, you could do a lot worse than dish up jacket potatoes (micro-waved, but crisped up in a hot oven for 10 minutes) with baked beans; pizzas made from a store-cupboard base with a tomato purée topping; a cheese omelette and salad, or scrambled eggs and mushrooms on toast.

Q: We seem to live on a menu loop of about five different meals at our house. What can I do to broaden their horizons?

🍅 Sally says: You're not alone. Many mums find themselves in the same sort of loop because, at the end of the day, you want to put something in front of them that they will actually eat rather than something you'll end up scraping into the bin. But it's really important to keep on trying new things if you want to expand their food horizons.

The trick is to take things steady and slow and build on what they do like – a whole new meal they've never seen before can lead to wrinkled noses and refusal among fussy eaters. So start by adding one new ingredient to an old favourite, such as grated carrot to bolognese, or a little curry powder into a casserole. Then you can progress to Quorn or turkey in the bolognese instead of beef or try turning it into a lasagne, or add a pastry or savoury crumble topping to the casserole to turn it into a pie.

It's worth continually searching for new options, from recipe books, on the internet, or among friends. Suggesting they join you in the kitchen while you cook can sometimes help to boost their interest in new meals.

Don't forget to encourage them to try something from your plate when you serve up something a little different for yourself. You never know – they might love it.

And finally, don't despair too much if you have a restricted menu at your house. As long as the limited choices you dish up represent a reasonable balance of foods, your kids will be fine. They're certain to become more adventurous as they grow.

Ten top tips for dealing with difficult eaters

We've condensed the most important points into 10 golden rules for dealing with difficult eaters. If you remember nothing else, remember these!

1. BE COOL

Easier said than done, admittedly, but it's true that attitude is everything when it comes to feeding children. Never let them see that their food issues are upsetting you – in some cases it will simply make things worse. In fact, don't let them upset you. It's okay. They'll survive – however bad it seems!

2. BE RESILIENT

Whether you're trying to expand the limited food horizons of a fussy eater, or overhaul the habits of a child with a weight problem, you'll need to be consistent, firm and resolute. You'll get there eventually. Hang in there.

3. BE A FOODIE

And encourage your kids to be, too. Get them in the kitchen, cooking their own food, and in the garden, growing it. Take them shopping, let them choose, allow them to prepare meals and snacks. Experiment, try something different every so often. And don't forget to talk about food – it's a fascinating subject.

4. BE A GOOD EATER YOURSELF

Sit at the table with them, eat your greens, and keep your treat intake limited. You are the foremost influence on your children, in eating and everything else. Their health is truly in your hands and the example you set is vital.

5. BE CAREFUL

Don't offer food as a bribe or reward, however desperate you get, and keep praise low-key. Be sure not to 'label' them – you may well have a difficult eater on your hands, but don't call them one to their face.

6. BE SENSITIVE

Watch out for the difficult eater with an underlying emotional need, and always treat the issue with care and understanding.

7. BE WELL INFORMED

Do your homework so you know what the basics of nutrition are – that way, you'll know off the top of your head what healthy alternatives you can offer a child who is asking for junk food; or an appropriate replacement when a child simply refuses to eat something. Bone up, too, on what makes children tick psychologically – understanding a situation always makes it easier to deal with it. And arm yourself with a good library of recipes and food ideas. There are so many different foods out there… it's just a matter of discovering them all.

8. BE UNITED

Get everyone else involved on your side. There's not much point in dealing with a difficult eater one way, if someone else is dealing with it a different way.

9. BE REASONABLE

Maybe your little difficult eater just doesn't like certain foods, or maybe they have a perfectly understandable preference for white bread. Why not? They may be kids, but they're also humans. A child should never be made to eat anything. Apart from being cruel, it's counter- productive and certainly won't make them more inclined to eat it in the future. And neither should a child be banished entirely from enjoying the things they love, sometimes.

10. BE MODERATE

Don't fret or obsess about food – apart from driving yourself insane, you may have the opposite effect to the one you were hoping for. What our kids eat is, and should be, something to care about and be concerned about. But leave it there. It's all about balance – as are most things in parenting. On one side of the scales sits the parent who doesn't give two hoots about their child's health (the sort who's prepared to shove a hamburger through a school gate because someone's made an effort to improve the school meal service, perhaps?) On the other is that mad old bat Muesli Mum, banning everything that's desirable, hovering over her children at every mealtime, and potentially creating the worst of attitudes towards eating in her child. Two extremes – the aim is to occupy the happy, healthy ground in the middle!

Useful contacts

Sources of information on general nutrition for children

www.food.gov.uk
Website of the Food Standards Agency, an independent Government department established to protect the public's health and consumer interests relating to food.

www.bda.uk.com
Website of the British Dietetic Association (BDA), the professional association for dietitians.

www.nutrition.org.uk
Website of the British Nutrition Foundation (BNF), a charity which aims to promote nutritional wellbeing.

www.vegsoc.org
Website of the Vegetarian Society, which includes nutritional information for families who don't eat meat.

Sources of information on weaning and feeding babies

www.netmums.com

Online community of mums which includes lots of useful information.

www.healthystart.nhs.uk

NHS site including weaning advice, plus information about free milk and food for families on benefits.

Sources of information on living a healthier lifestyle

www.nhs.uk/change4life

Website of Change4life, an NHS campaign promoting healthier lifestyles for modern families.

www.shape-up.org

Website of Weight Concern, a charity set up to tackle the rise of obesity.

www.weightlossresources.co.uk

Website offering a vast array of nutritional and diet information for all age groups, including children and young people.

Sources of information about dietary special needs

www.hacsg.org.uk
Website of the Hyperactive Children's Support Group.

www.actiononadditives.com
Website of the Action on Additives campaign.

www.kidsallergies.co.uk
Website offering comprehensive information about children and allergies.

www.foodsmatter.com
Independent site with lots of information on food allergies and intolerances.

Where to find an independent dietitian or nutritionist

www.dietitiansunlimited.co.uk
Website run by the British Dietetic Association's freelance dietitian group.

www.bant.org.uk
Website of the British Association of Nutrional Therapists.

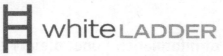

whiteLADDER

the parenting & family health experts

Get 30% off your next purchase...

We are publishers of a growing **parenting and family health** range of books. We pride ourselves on our friendly and accessible approach whilst providing you with sensible, non-preachy information. This is what makes us **different from other publishers**.

And we are keen to **find out what you think** about our book.

If you love this book **tell us why** and tell your friends. And if you think we could do better, **let us know**. Your thoughts and opinions are important to us and help us produce the best books we possibly can.

As a **thank you** we'll give you 30% off your next purchase. Write to us at **info@whiteladderpress.co.uk** and we'll send you an online voucher by return.

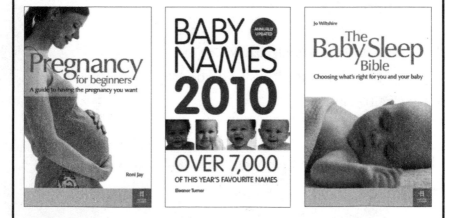

Come and visit us at **www.whiteladderpress.co.uk**